I0090466

THE
CAT SAFETY
BIBLE

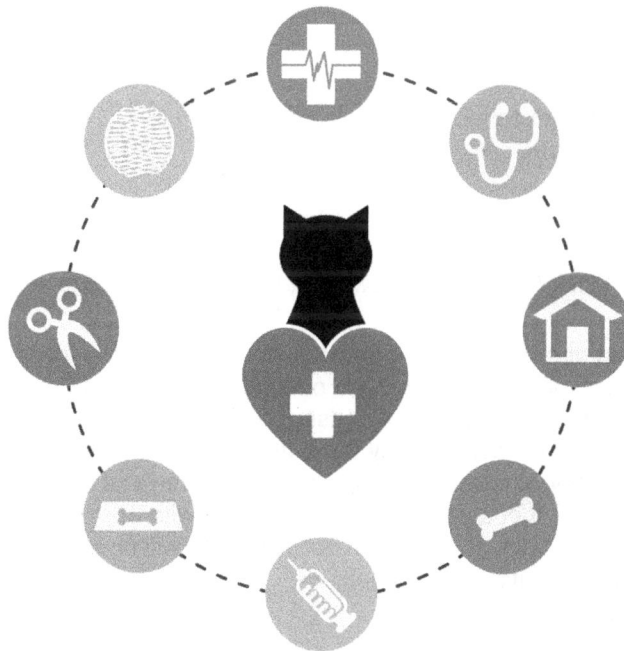

**Pet Safety and First Aid
For Your Cat**

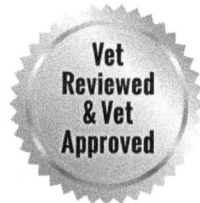

Vet
Reviewed
& Vet
Approved

DENISE FLECK and ROBERT SEMROW

Important Note Regarding Cat Care,
First-Aid & CPCR Techniques Provided In This Book

*If you have any questions about your cat's health,
seek professional Veterinary care immediately!*

*These recommendations and the contents of this book are designed
to help you keep your cat more comfortable and aid with minor problems before
you are able to get to (or are on your way to) an animal hospital or Veterinarian's office.*

They are not meant to be a substitute for care by a licensed Veterinary professional.

*No liability is assumed by the authors, publisher or any other party with respect
to the information, suggestions and techniques described in this book.*

*Should there be any discrepancy between the suggestions offered
and the advice of a Veterinarian, it is recommended that the advice
of the Veterinarian be followed since the Veterinarian has the advantage
of physically examining the cat and knowing its medical history and circumstances.*

Published by Pet World Media Group
4533 Mac Arthur Blvd. #340, Newport Beach, CA 92660
E-Mail: Info@petworldmediagroup.com
Phone: 888-969-7297

Copyright © 2019 Denise Fleck / Robert Semrow / Pet World Media Group

All rights reserved. No part of this publication may be reproduced in any form without the
written permission of the copyright owners and the publisher. All images in this book have
been reproduced with the knowledge and prior consent of the artists, individuals and agencies
concerned, and no responsibility is accepted by the authors, publisher, producers, or printer for
any infringement of copyright or otherwise, arising from the contents of this publication. Every
effort has been made to ensure that credits accurately comply with the information supplied.
We apologize for any inaccuracies that may have occurred and will fix inaccurate or missing
information in a subsequent reprinting of the book.

ISBN: 978-1-949695-10-6

First Edition

Printed and Manufactured in the United States of America

Information and updates on this book and other Pet World Media Group projects
can be found on www.petworldmediagroup.com

Paperback - Black & White Course Workbook
Edition

TABLE OF CONTENTS

Section Two: Why You Should Know Cat First-Aid & CPCR

Important Note Regarding Cat Care, First Aid & CPCR Techniques Provided In This Book

If you have any questions about your Cat's health, seek professional Veterinary care immediately!

These recommendations and the contents of this book are designed to help you keep your pet more comfortable and aid with minor problems before you are able to get to (or are on your way to) an animal hospital or Veterinarian's office.

They are not meant to be a substitute for care by a licensed Veterinary professional.

No liability is assumed by the authors, publisher or any other party with respect to the information, suggestions and techniques described in this book.

Should there be any discrepancy between the suggestions offered and the advice of a Veterinarian, it is recommended that the advice of the Veterinarian be followed since the Veterinarian has the advantage of physically examining the cat and knowing its medical history and circumstances.

Published by Pet World Media Group
4533 Mac Arthur Blvd. #340, Newport Beach, CA 92660
E-Mail: Info@petworldmediagroup.com
Phone: 888-969-7297

Copyright © 2019 Denise Fleck / Robert Semrow / Pet World Media Group

All rights reserved. No part of this publication may be reproduced in any form without the written permission of the copyright owners and the publisher. All images in this book have been reproduced with the knowledge and prior consent of the artists, individuals and agencies concerned, and no responsibility is accepted by the authors, publisher, producers, or printer for any infringement of copyright or otherwise, arising from the contents of this publication. Every effort has been made to ensure that credits accurately comply with the information supplied. We apologize for any inaccuracies that may have occurred and will fix inaccurate or missing information in a subsequent reprinting of the book.

ISBN: 978-1-949695-10-6

Printed and Manufactured in the United States of America

Information and updates on this book and other Pet World Media Group projects can be found on www.petworldmediagroup.com

BEFORE YOU ADOPT

Sharing your life with a cat may be one of the most rewarding things you ever do during your lifetime…it totally ROCKS, but…it is a HUGE responsibility! Another living being will depend on you for its entire life, and YOU must make that life as safe and satisfying as possible. No matter what curves life throws your way, how much you change, get busy or tired, even if your income declines, you must keep your heart, schedule and home open for the cat you have made part of your family for its lifetime!

Caring for a four-legged friend takes time, money and energy, so you must be committed, willing to work hard and even make a compromise along the way to be a good cat parent.

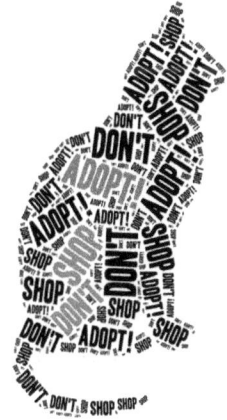

CHOOSING YOUR CAT

Felis catis are small furry carnivorous mammals we call house cats as they share our lives and the indoors with us. We value them for their companionship and ability to hunt rodents. Not all cats look or act the same. Some are active, some are couch potatoes, others like to sit quietly in your lap and purr loudly while others roam the premises vocalizing at the top of their kitty cat lungs. The Cat Fanciers Association (CFA) & The International Cat Association (TICA) recognize more than 70 different breeds of felines, but of course, there are mixed breeds as well. In addition to breed characteristics, each cat has his or her own unique personality. However, some generalizations can be made to help you better choose the one best suited for you.

In the cat world, the American Shorthair is even-tempered and quiet while the Abyssinian is more active. The Burmese has a short coat and is very people friendly. The tail-less Manx is quiet and gentle. If you're looking for a large cat, the Maine Coon fits the bill and as a rule, he is good with both kids and dogs. The Sphynx is hair-less (well she does have a little fuzz) while the sleek Siamese can be quite vocal. Ragdolls are docile but have long coats that need constant brushing or you'll end up having to get a professional to shave the mats off. Long-coated cats require more grooming, so that is more time and work for you but can be so rewarding. Additionally, if you don't "brush the kitty, brush the kitty," she will ingest hair grooming herself which can result in troublesome fur balls. If you don't comb out your cat, she could get matted which can lead to uncomfortable sores and ultimately cause her to have to be shaved down at the groomers.

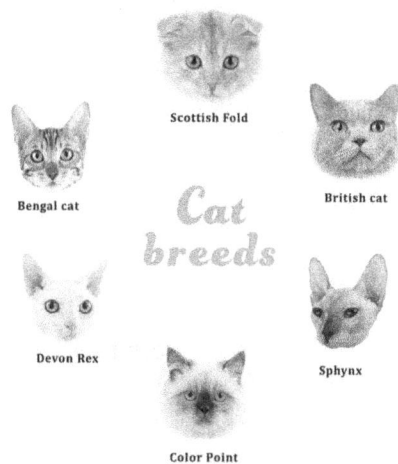

Scottish Fold

Bengal cat

British cat

Cat breeds

Devon Rex

Sphynx

Color Point

Kittens need to be litter trained. Will you gladly get up every two hours during the night for feedings and bathroom breaks? Can you sleep through the incessant cries coming from the tiny furry creature who wants nothing more than to be cuddled by you at 3am? And maybe those cries shouldn't be ignored, so will you get up and see what is ailing your tiny kitten? How about those wet spots on the carpet (or the middle of your bed) until Fluffy learns to use the litter box? Kittens don't know the rules and require a patient human to teach them. When you adopt a small furry friend you must be prepared for sleepless nights, rushing home to check on them and remain equipped with lots and lots of endless love. Senior cats have it down…they know their manners, are calmer and even more focused. They are often perfectly content to let you go about your day lying by your side (or in your lap), thrilled for a pat on the head or the occasional ear scratch. They just want to be with you, but as time goes by, they may require medical care. Is your bank account prepared for that? Patience again becomes of prime importance as accidents happen when cats get older. You will need to develop ways to make clean-up easier so that you never lose your temper with your best feline. Ideas are discussed later in this book.

Ask yourself:

- How much time can you spend with your cat each day? Cats do better at home alone.
- Where will your cat be while you are at work, school or running errands? In a crate, one room or have free roam of the house?
- Do you have a catio or secure "cat fencing" if she has access to the outdoors. You certainly don't want your cat to jump out of your fence, but you also don't want another animal to jump or swoop in and capture her!
- Where will you place the kitty's bed, bowls and toys so that they are not in the way but safely positioned?
- Can your budget accommodate an animal's basic needs? Food, bed, collar, toys, micro-chipping, spay/neuter, veterinary exams, flea/tick prevention, and the unexpected.
- How much time can you spend grooming? Even with a groomer, you need to do daily maintenance and a good head-to-tail check-up weekly (see page 37)!
- Will you be able to take care of your new best friend no matter what? If you move, add another family member (young or old), get a new job, go off to college, have a change in health or income, what will happen to your four legged family member?

Other Considerations:

Apartment Dweller?

People who want to share their life with a cat are lucky as they work well in small spaces, however if your cat is going to be left alone, he may mew, meow and even howl. Take this into consideration if you share walls with a neighbor. Also, cats do need exercise and will run and bounce about. That might be a consideration if you have a neighbor living on a floor beneath you. Good pet parents make good neighbors!

Landlord Restrictions?

Cats, and be specific with the species, don't just ask if pets are allowed. Although it is even more likely that your landlord will be agreeable to you having a feline roommate, some have had bad experiences, unable to remove cat urine from carpets, so that may not be as understanding. Find out upfront before you rent.

Local Laws?

Some jurisdictions only allow a certain number of cats per household (a combination of three dogs or cats for instance), so check with your local animal control before you adopt. Unfortunately, some cities ban specific breeds. Others may place restrictions on them (such as they must be spayed/neutered, or cannot roam certain areas). You are not only your cat's advocate, but you are also his protector and must know how to keep him safe as well as law-abiding.

Yard/Fencing?

The number of pets hit by cars every year is staggering. There are no guarantees, but most indoor-only cats live much longer lives and thrive. If your cat enjoys the fresh air and sunshine, a securely screened porch is a great option but there is also cat fencing that prevents her from hopping over. Do note however, that although your cat may not be able to leave her enclosed yard, other animals, including birds of prey, may be able to enter. An enclosed catio is truly the best option.

Cats that don't roam the neighborhood also avoid:
- Pesticides on your neighbor's lawn
- Poisons in garbage cans
- Fights with other animals

Indoor Cats vs. Outdoor Cats?

Although some people wrongly assume it is cruel to keep a cat in the house all day, indoor cats are less likely to be exposed to viruses, don't get into poisons found in the neighbor's garbage, avoid getting hit by cars, attacked by wildlife or even the dog next door. According to numerous surveys, many outdoors cats live only 2-5 years while their indoor counterparts generally thrive for 10-15 years, or even more! Chances are your indoor cat won't pick up fleas or ticks either. Ultimately, an indoor cat's biggest problem may be boredom, but that can be alleviated with toys, another cat and time spent with YOU! It just makes good safety sense to protect your cat by keeping her indoors. If kitty enjoys fresh air beyond the screened porch, special fencing that attaches to your chain link angling inward 45° can prevent her from roaming but may

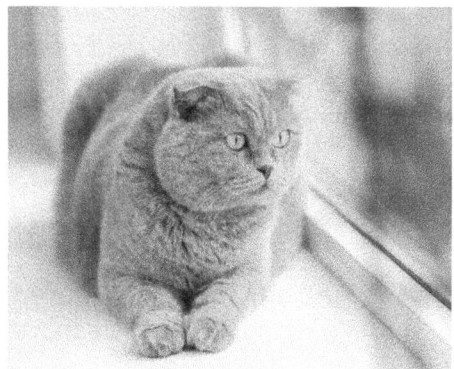

not prevent predators from getting in. Human supervision is always an important component. Also be diligent checking window screens making sure your sun-worshiping feline can't push it loose and topple to the ground from an upstairs sill. Cats do not always land on their feet and are often injured (see page 159 in the First-Aid Section on Falls & High-rise injuries).

Children?

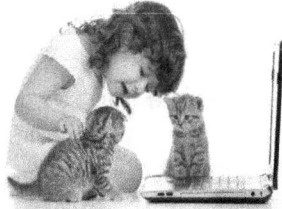

Cats can sometimes become overwhelmed by the smallest of humans and hiss, snarl, scratch and bite. can sometimes become overwhelmed by the smallest humans and act snippy. Supervise ALL animals around children, and teach children not to disturb a cat while it is sleeping, eating or playing with its toys.

Both children and cas can be unpredictable and leaving them alone together without adult supervision could be a recipe for disaster. You must take charge and be there to intercede rather than trusting an animal or child to always do the right thing.

Allergies to Cats?

Don't rule out adding a cat to the family. Being around pets can strengthen the immune system (See "Zooeyia" on page 5) but do check with your physician to see if there are medications to keep you comfortable should you get watery eyes, a runny nose or a case of the sneezes. Give it time, but vacuum the house regularly and bathe the cat frequently. This may take patience but is worth the love you will share.. More people seem to be bothered by cat dander but again, every animal and person are different so bring home a towel the cat has slept on for a few days. If you're not in distress with her scent around, you might have found the perfect new friend!

Other Pets?

Introduce your cat slowly and carefully to other animals in the household. Just because you want one big happy family doesn't mean all animals will immediately (or ever) get along. Provide an out-of-claws-reach location for pocket pets, fish and birds which look like prey animals to many felines.

There are always exceptions, but generally the following combinations work best in a MULTIPLE CAT HOUSEHOLD:

- Two kittens
- An adult neutered/spayed cat and a kitten
- Two adult neutered/spayed cats (either two females or a male and a female)

The most volatile combination seems to be two non-neutered mature male cats.

Always consider your current cat's personality before introducing a new cat. An active cat is more likely to accept a new kitten while a quieter, more reclusive cat might prefer a mature adult as a companion. See page 32 for ways to introduce your cat to a new friend.

If you're considering adding a adding a cat to your canine pack, patience and caution are key! Read through the INTRODUCTIONS section on page 32 in this book, get advice from the shelter you adopt from and supervise, supervise, supervise. There just are no hard and fast rules.

Zooeyia?

Are you tilting your head like a confused feline about now? Zooeyia (ZOO-ey-ah) is a relatively new word which describes the health benefits pets provide us humans! It comes from the Greek roots "zoion" for animal and "Hygeia" for the Greek goddess of health, and its inventors consider it the opposite of Zoonosis which you'll read about on page 51. Zoonosis refers to diseases that can be transferred between species, meaning ones you can get from your pets.

Science is proving that making a pet part of your family can decrease the risk of developing colds and asthma by developing stronger immune systems. Pets lower our stress and also our blood pressure, but there are other health issues recently identified by the Institute of Medicine of the National Academies:

- Pets get us moving.
- Pets lower the impact of chronic disease. Studies have shown cats decrease the risk of cardiovascular disease in their owners. Having a pet in the life of a cancer patient has been shown to provide comfort and support during treatment, which can decrease stress and releases endorphins.
- Pets help us kick the habit. Research has shown that knowing secondhand smoke can harm our pets has motivated some smokers to quit!
- Pets make us more social. Loneliness and isolation can occur in our increasingly urbanized lifestyles, especially among the elderly. Having a pet gets us out meeting people, taking part in activities with other pet parents, going to parks, hiking and just staying in touch with the world.

Do your research, and make a well thought out decision before you adopt, and then embrace the joys of having a pet as part of the family! Not only will you have a furry friend who loves you unconditionally, but also look at all the other ways he may benefit your health as well.

WHERE TO MEET YOUR NEW CAT?

Local Animal Shelters take in 3 - 4 million dogs and cats each year. A common myth is that shelters only have mixed breeds, but it is simply not true! In most cases, 25% are purebreds, and the rest are amazing animals too. Visit several times and spend time interacting with the kitty of your choice before deciding. Do not choose through a window or kennel door alone.

Many humans feel that rescue pets are particularly grateful for being saved, but if you are looking for a specific breed that you can't find at your local shelter, breed-specific rescue organizations can be found on-line.

Responsible breeders take their jobs of raising dogs seriously. You'll know they are responsible not only by the care given and the depth of their knowledge, but they also will agree to take back the animal at any time during his life if you are unable to care for him. To locate a responsible breeder, contact the Cat Fanciers Association (CFA), The International Cat Association (TICA) or other reputable organization.

SATISFYING YOUR CAT'S BASIC NEEDS

Get off on the right paw with your new best friend by fulfilling her basic needs for a longer, happier lifetime together:

1) Quality Time Spent with You
2) Supplies
3) Health & Safety Team
4) Identification
5) Nutrition
6) Exercise & Stretching, Socialization & Basic Manners
7) Educate yourself for your cat's sake

1) <u>Quality Time Spent with YOU</u>

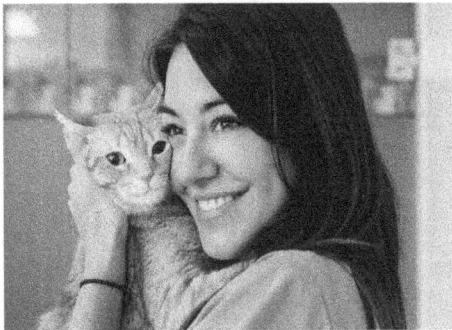

The true meaning of life for your cat is quality time spent with their favorite person -- YOU! Feline lives are much shorter than ours, so make every minute count and live in the moment with your precious pet. Take time out to do special activities together, such as grooming, ear scratches, laying in the sun together or getting involved in agility...whatever makes you smile and your kitty purr! Get involved in agility (cats too are now taking up this sport), or chasing a feather -- whatever makes you smile and your kitty purr!

2) Supseline

- Bed
- Bowls
- Brush, Comb, Flea Comb
- Carrier/Crate
- Collar
- Cat License (where applicable)
- Flea & Tick Prevention
- Food
- Pet Toothbrush & Pet Specific Toothpaste
- ID Tag that is clearly legible & Microchip properly registered & maintained
- Necessary medication/supplements
- Cat First-Aid Kit
- Cat Sitter when you can't be there
- Plan for her care if you are injured
- Toys
- Training/Behaviorist
- Veterinary Care/Insurance
- Unexpected Expenses

3) Your Cat's Health & Safety Team (aka her body guards, entourage, people)

Through research and conversation with other cat parents and professionals, you must assemble a team to care for your pet. The primary caregivers, also known as your cat's 'second best friends' (well you are #1 after all), should include your Veterinarian, Emergency Center Personnel, Groomer and Cat Sitter. You could need to add to the team depending on your lifestyle or cat's needs, so those humans may include: Boarding or Daycare Staff, Animal Behaviorist, Animal Communicator, Holistic Veterinarian, Massage Therapist, Acupuncturist and/or Nutritionist along with various medical specialists. Additionally, you should designate at least 2-3 people who could care for your cat in the event you are unable to and have paper work in order to make sure your wishes are honored. (See form on page 216).

Veterinarian

Consider your Veterinarian's qualifications, but also:

- Location, office hours, payment options, range of services
- Can you get an appointment quickly?
- Is your Veterinarian's philosophy and openness to alternative treatments in line with your own beliefs?
- Does the Veterinarian have a good bedside manner and answer questions to your satisfaction? Knowledge and expertise is a wonderful thing, but since you speak for your cat who cannot, you must put together a team of humans that YOU and your cat can relate to and build a good rapport with. Is there a separate cat-friendly entrance and or waiting area and is the veterinarian certified in Fear Free® techniques?

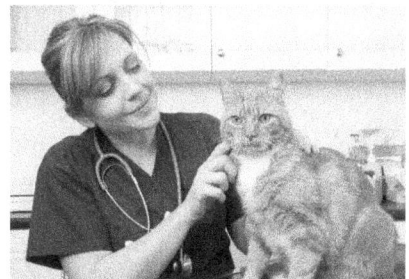

Ask friends if they like their Veterinarian and notice:
- If the office is clean
- If the waiting room accommodates multiple pets
- If the front office staff is helpful and tends to stay
- If they are a member of the American Animal Hospital Association (AAHA) which means they have met certain standards.
- The office environment and the interactions of staff, noting if people and pets are treated in a manner you are comfortable with, if there are safe waiting areas and if the general care and vibe fits your needs.

Bring your pet to the Veterinarian for
- Annual check-ups
- Vaccinations
- Spay/Neuter
  Unaltered pets roam in search of a mate and 80% of animals killed on highways are non-neutered males. Animals that aren't "fixed" often display a higher level of aggression and are at greater risk for pyometra, mammary and prostate cancers. With 3 - 4 million homeless animals being euthanized each year, become part of the solution, not part of the problem.
- Senior exams including blood panel and urinalysis
- Anytime your cat is not quite right.

Animal Emergency Center

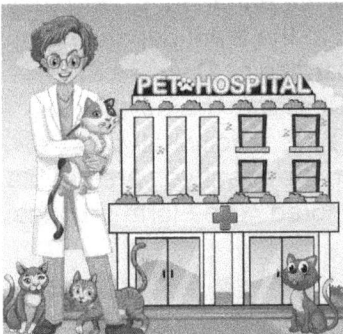

Some are open 24/7 while others keep the hours your Veterinarian is closed…6pm – 8am the next morning. Find the one nearest your home, your favorite park or hiking location and wherever your dog goes and DRIVE THERE! Writing down the address and phone number is not enough. When an emergency happens you must be on auto-pilot and know where you are headed for your cat's sake.

Must Know:
- Where the office is located
- Where to park
- Is there a separate entrance for cats.
- What services can be provided – Is the facility equipped for x-rays, MRIs, transfusions, surgeries? Do they carry antivenin for snake bites? Do your research and be prepared before you need to help your pet.
- Payment options

Whether an emergency or routine care, veterinary insurance could help you help your cat when your bank account cannot. Check into the various options and restrictions, researching which plan is best for you and the current cat in your life. Deductibles and procedures covered vary from policy to policy. Should you opt not to purchase insurance, you may be preventing your pet from getting much-needed care, so have a Plan B! At the very least, have an emergency credit card or a separate bank account that you contribute to monthly in the event your furry loved one needs medical care.

Obedience Trainer

This could be YOU, but ALL cats need to learn basic obedience to become welcomed members of the family! "Come" or "Stay" can help your cat stay out of harm's way. "Leave it" could prevent her from ingesting poison! Humans have boundaries and do best when courteous so our four-legged companions must be taught to do the same for a happy and safe lifetime together.

As the adage goes, dogs have owners and cats have staff, but learning can take place if you practice together daily throughout your cat's lifetime. You CAN teach an older cat new tricks…keep her mind sharp and you engaged in her life.

Groomer

Most people think of this team member as the beautician, but there is much more to a groomer than the fur on your cat! The groomer, even more than your Veterinarian, gets down to your cat's skin and can notice eruptions, cuts, scrapes, allergies and rashes. Your groomer may find a bump while bathing your cat or notice your dog's ears are infected. Choose your groomer well, and he or she may be your catt's first line of defense in finding a problem before it becomes a nightmare.

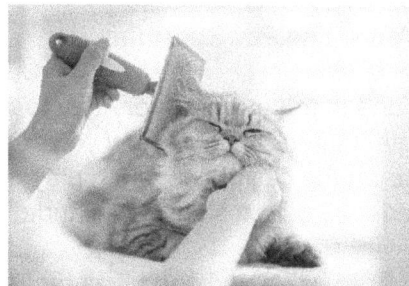

Cat Sitter

Although the enthusiastic neighboorhood teen who loves your cat may be a good choice to watch him or her when you're away, please hire a professional pet sitter for your fur kid. The person caring for your best friend must take the responsibility to heart and seriously prepare to handle whatever life throws their way when caring for a precious life. Your cat's sitter should be licensed, bonded and able to anticipate a situation BEFORE it arises with the confidence to handle it. Yes, you want a true blue animal person who will greet your cat, maybe even before he or she greets you, but also one who can read animal body language and observe mood changes. You also need someone who can carefully place kitty in and out of her carrier, administer medications and has cat centric knowledge. Someone who will follow your directions to a tee. Knowledge, experience and dependability are key traits to seek out in your cat's caregiver.

Just as you are learning from this book, a professional pet sitter keeps on learning better ways to relate to and care for animals, can safely administer Pet First-Aid & CPCR and must know what to do if the power goes out or a pipe breaks when you are away -- For your pet's sake. A professional pet sitter prides him or herself on staying current on all things pet -- the latest in nutrition, exercise, safety and care, so they are an excellent resource for you as well. Seeking a recommendation from other conscientious pet parents or your Veterinarian (many Vet techs pet sit on the side) is a GRRReat choice, but professional organizations, such as Pet Sitters International™, can provide you with a list of certified professional pet sitters in your area. PSI and NAPPS (National Association of Professional Pet Sitters) provide on-line and in-person trainings to their members, provide excellent guidelines to keep them organized with their sits and motivate them to be the best pet caregiver they can be.

Once you have chosen a reliable pet sitter, make sure you put into place any authorizations needed on your pet's behalf, so that the pet sitter may obtain necessary care for your cat in your absence. Put everything in writing that your pet's caregiver should know including medical history, food, places pet sleeps and hide. Fill in your Pet's Health Record on page 247, and you'll be set. Talk with your Veterinarian's office to determine if a letter is required (and possibly your credit card) to be kept on file to allow your pet sitter to make medical decisions for your pet if you are not reachable. Discuss this also with your cat sitter, so that he or she knows to what extent you want medical care for your pets and who you want providing treatment for them.

You – The Pet Guardian

Tune in to your cat every day to notice subtle changes and stay in-the-know to get the latest information on how you can help your pet live a longer, happier healthier life! Don't be on the cell phone when playing with Fluffy -- give her your undivided attention for at least 20 minutes each day and even more time just spent near or with you.

Be proactive and don't wait for tragedy to strike. Keep a simple Identification Card (like you'll find on page 216) in your wallet to let first responders know you have pets at home that need caring for if something happens to you. Can you imagine your poor kitty distressed over a dirty litter box or wondering when you'll be home to feed her if you haven't made this plan? Besides filling out the paperwork, you MUST be sure that caregivers you designate are totally on board and know how you'd like your cat cared for. Include funds for them to do so. Hopefully this care will just be short term, but it is wise to meet with an attorney and put everything in writing. Publish this document, making sure others know it exists and that these are your wishes. This should NOT be part of your Will as it could need to be enacted while you are still alive, such as if you are in a coma or suffer some other disability that will not permit you to care for your best friends. Don't let your fur kids be relinquished or sent off to a Shelter because you didn't take the time to plan for them. You can't assume family members will make them their own. Get everything legally prepared and confirm with all parties involved. Also designate at least three caregivers as circumstances in their own lives may have changed when they are needed most.

4) Identification Should Include

- Cat's name
- Your name, address, telephone numbers
- Medical problem(s) requiring medication
- Veterinarian's name & number
- Current rabies vaccination information
- Reward offer which increases chances your cat will be returned to you

Microchips are important as tags can fall off. A microchip is a tiny electronic chip enclosed in a glass cylinder (about the size of a grain of rice) that is injected just under your cat's skin – between his shoulder blades – with a hypodermic needle. The microchip does not have a battery but is activated when a scanner is passed over your pet. It transmits an ID number to the scanner along with the name of the microchip's manufacturer. If you have done your homework and sent the registering agency your contact information, your pet's microchip will identify them as belonging to you.

Microchips are a safe and effective way to reunite pets with their humans – they are also used on dogs, birds, horses, rabbits, and just about any pet.

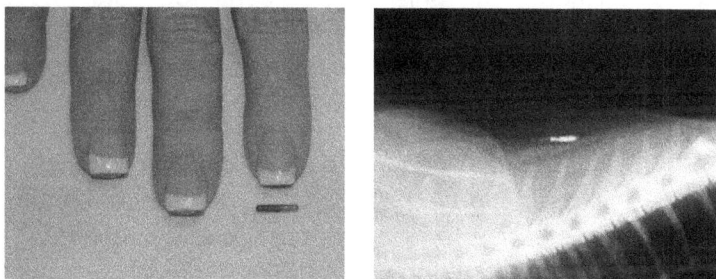

Photos Courtesy of Sunny-dog Ink

Check tags regularly to insure information is legible and accurate.

If your kitty wears a collar and tags, many indoor cats do not, check to make sure engraving hasn't rubbed off and is easy to read. Also have your cat scanned during his annual veterinary visit to make sure the microchip is still in place (they can migrate in your cat's body) and working as it should. Update contact information with your microchip company when you move or change a phone number, and check with your local animal shelter to make sure they use a universal scanner that reads your microchip. If not, encourage them to get one that does or make sure your pets have microchips that can be read by your local facility.

Good to Know:

The International Standards Organization (ISO) has approved a global standard for microchips which is intended to create a consistent ID system worldwide. For example, if your cat is implanted with an ISO standard microchip in the U.S. travels to Europe with you and becomes lost, the ISO standard scanners in Europe would be able to read the microchip. If your dog however was implanted with a non-ISO microchip, it might not be detected or be read by the scanner.

Should your pet ever go missing:

Contact your microchip company, Veterinarian and local shelter at once. Make flyers using a current photo and stating a reward (it definitely increases the chances of re-uniting you with your best friend) and circulate them all over the neighborhood taking care to abide by city rules as to where and how you may post. Walk the neighborhood asking if anyone has seen your cat and visit local shelters as well as various websites with data bases that list found pets.

Hire one of the many services out there that will make robo-calls to your entire neighborhood and get your cat's photo on numerous websites and social media to increase the possibility of a safe return. There are trained Pet Detectives, some even use dogs to find your pet, so get acquainted with the various help available to help your cat find her way home. ("Missing Cat" flyer template on page 214)

5) Nutrition: Take a More Active Role in Your Cat's Diet and Health by Choosing the Best Food for Your Cat

"You are what you eat." Although this phrase has a contrived history dating back centuries, it didn't emerge in English until 1940 when nutritionist Victor Lindlahr wrote the book so entitled expressing his strong belief that food controls health. It holds true for our feline friends too.

Most consumers are unaware that the pet food industry got its early start as an opportunity to sell off waste from the human food industry. Shocking but true, contaminated and low quality sources of meat (animal by-products) that are rejected by the USDA (United States Department of Agriculture) can be sold to pet food companies at bargain prices. These discarded ingredients may include intestines, udders, heads, hooves and even diseased and cancerous animal parts. But there is good news! "Fortunately, more progressive pet food companies are rejecting the use of inferior meat and grain by-products, are accepting only USDA-inspected meats, and are not adding artificial flavorings and unnatural preservatives to their new diets," says Paula Terifaj, DVM in Brea, California. Therefore, one of the best things you can do for your cat is to know what you are feeding him. To do so you must read and understand pet food labels and research the brand you buy.

BCCF (Before Commercial Cat Food)

Less than a hundred years ago, the family pet ate leftovers and table scraps in addition to scavenging and hunting. Whether pets truly thrived on this diet is hard to say according to Deb Eldredge, DVM in Vernon, New York. "We keep better records now and have better diagnostics."

INCREASED AWARENESS

The move towards healthier eating by people shows in the concern over our cat's diet as well. Susan Blake Davis, a Certified Clinical Nutritionist who provides holistic pet health consultations nationwide claims, "Many health-minded pet owners want the same high quality food for their pets that they eat themselves. While many are preparing homemade foods, others are demanding that the same quality be found in commercially prepared foods that are convenient and easy to use. As a result, there are lots of wonderful brands on the market." However, Dr. Terifaj cautions not to be fooled by claims that pet foods labeled 'balanced and nutritionally complete' really are. "You are in a dangerous comfort zone if you believe that any one diet can be formulated [to be complete for every pet.]" Each cat, like every individual human, is different with varying genetics, environments, sensitivities and needs. No one diet is perfect for all. Cats out of the same litter may not thrive on the same diet.

Additionally, the Menu Foods Recall of 2007 brought to light the fact that store bought pet food isn't always safe and can be life-threatening. "With commercially prepared food," explains Dr. Eldredge, "pets are now getting a more balanced diet. In the past Veterinarians saw more cases of vitamin deficiencies or excesses, yet on the other hand, with the mass production of food, if a contaminated ingredient gets into the diet, we have large numbers of pets throughout a wide area being affected."

The 2007 Recall wasn't the first but it was the largest. In 1998 fifty-three brands of pet food were found to be contaminated with aflatoxin (a toxin produced by mold that can damage the liver) and ten more brands in 2005. There were other recalls prior and more have and will follow, so pet parents need to take a more active role in the health of their pets.

Ignore packaging and clever names. Look at the actual ingredients. Much of the commercial food available today is made for the benefit of the consumer. It is made to be convenient, colorful and attractive. Orange carrot-shaped treats give consumers the false sense that they are giving their pet a real carrot. Remember that Mother Nature gives us our most basic rules: *Eat fresh, choose variety and buy wholesome.*

Must-know Vocabulary as determined by the AAFCO (Association of American Food Control Officials)...

Meat is "the clean flesh derived from slaughtered mammals and is limited to that part of the striate muscle which is skeletal or that which is found in the tongue, diaphragm, heart or esophagus."

Poultry is "the clean combination of flesh and skin with or without accompanying bone, derived from the parts or whole carcasses of poultry or a combination thereof, exclusive of feathers, heads, feet and entrails."

Meal is the rendered product from mammal tissues, exclusive of any added blood, hair, feathers, hooves, horn, hide, trimmings, manure, stomach and rumen contents except in such amounts as may occur unavoidably."

By Product consists of "non-rendered clean parts of carcasses free from fecal content and foreign matter."

MBM aka Meat and Bone Meal is a catch-all term where the worst stories come from about pet food. Some renderers accept road kill, euthanized pets, animals who died on farms, during transport, fetuses and out-of-date supermarket meat so MBM is a signal that the food is of inferior quality for your best friend.

Basic Guidelines:

- The first two ingredients should be whole sources of specific animal protein: beef, chicken, lamb, salmon, venison, turkey or other animal protein...The name of the animal in the bag or can. Stay away from the terms "meat," "poultry" and "fish" which are too vague.
- Whenever possible limit or avoid meat & filler by-products as well as fillers (wheat, corn and soy for instance which can cause allergies or are hard for pets to process).
- Stay away from food dyes, sweeteners such as propylene glycol and sorbitol, additives like smoke or beef flavor and sodium nitrite which all carry health risks.
- As a rule, canned food is preferable to dry for cats as they suffer less urinary tract and kidney problems when consuming food that has water in it.
- Avoid artificial preservatives (BHA, BHT and ethoxyquin), and seek out foods using natural antioxidants like vitamins C, E and mixed tocopherols. Frozen foods avoid the use of unnatural preservatives altogether since freezing naturally preserves food.
- Educate yourself as to which human foods are unsafe for your pet. Two good sources are www.aspca.org and www.hsus.org.

Specifically for Cats:

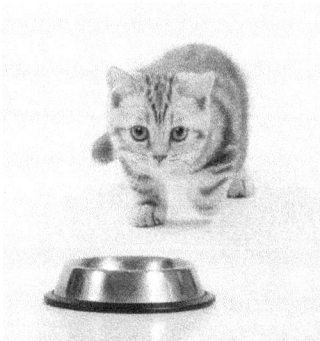

Rule #1 Cats are TRUE carnivores and require meat in their diet daily, but they are not the best water drinkers, so they often suffer from urinary problems. Therefore, meat in a canned or other wet form is often their best diet.

Rule #2 Cats cannot produce TAURINE, an essential amino acid found in animal products. Taurine deficiency can result in improper fetal development, blindness and/or a weakening of the heart muscle among other health issues. Tuna DOES NOT have a significant amount of taurine, so a diet of tuna alone can be harmful to your cat!

Rule #3 More and more cats are developing allergies to fish and chicken, so if your kitty is red, itchy or not quite right, start eliminating one ingredient at a time from her diet to determine if the symptoms could be food related.

Realize that pet food is distributed and sold in various ways – chain pet stores, independent stores and via the internet, so you won't find all brands in one location. Make time to explore your options for the health of your cat. Foods loaded with fillers (corn, meal, gluten) require more food to make a cat feel full. Additionally, a cat thriving on a nutritious diet will spend less time running up a tab at your Veterinarian's office.

Finding the right diet depends upon the unique needs of your pet, and maybe…even each of your pets. Cats born in the same litter may not respond well on the same diet. The right diet depends upon your pet's age, weight and health conditions.

Carbohydrates can be beneficial for certain health conditions such as liver disease, but in a young healthy dog or cat, excessive carbs can lead to yeast overgrowth and allergy issues. Pets on a poor diet may show weight gain or loss, poor coats, less than ideal growth or bone problems.

The best diet for any pet is the diet that pet does best on.

Pay attention to the sparkle in your pet's eyes, his energy level, coat condition and passion for life. Have your cat tested for any deficiencies or diseases that could be improved by a proper diet. A few more dollars spent on more nutritious food can reduce veterinary visits and improve the health of your four-legged best friend. That is truly priceless!

Label Reading 101

There's no way around it. To be a responsible cat parent, you must learn to read pet food labels to avoid buying an inferior product for your feline best friend. Some higher priced foods also contain undesirable ingredients, so don't be fooled by the price tag or marketing campaign. Clever advertising gurus try to seduce you with photos of succulent meats and vegetables and happy animal faces. Don't judge any pet food by its wrapper!

Ingredients are listed in descending order of weight, and animal protein is the single most important ingredient in pet food, so look at the first few ingredients listed to determine the main sources of protein being used. Pay attention if other items are broken into components -- if chicken is listed first, but then comes corn gluten, corn meal and ground corn, those three corn components may add up to a higher concentration than the chicken.

Equally important as what you want to see on the label, are those items you do not want to see – chemical additives and preservatives. Below is a brief glossary of labeling "buzz" words to familiarize yourself with:

All or 100% cannot be used (according to AAFCO guidelines) "if the product contains more than one ingredient, not including water sufficient for processing, [includes anything that colors substandard meats to look more natural], or trace amounts of preservatives and condiments]."

95% Rule applies when the ingredients derived from animals, poultry or fish make up 95% or more of the total weight of the product (or 70% excluding water for processing).

Flavor means the ingredients impart a distinctive characteristic to the food. Therefore, a "beef flavor" food may contain a small quantity of digest (material which results from a chemical or enzymatic process) or other extract of tissues or artificial flavor, without containing any actual beef meat at all.

Guaranteed analysis provides a very general guide to the composition of the food. Crude protein, fat, fiber and total moisture are required to be listed. Beware that the term crude protein allows pet food manufacturers to include items such as feathers, hair, hooves, tendons, and ligaments in their diets. While these animal by-products certainly contain protein, they are essentially indigestible and provide no nutritional value to your cat.

Holistic has yet to be embraced by regulations and standards with regards to pet food, so any manufacturer can claim the phrase on their packaging.

Human grade can be misleading unless the entire product is edible by humans, in accordance to USDA and FDA standards.

Organic means USDA rules and regulations must be followed and the product will have the USDA organic seal on the packaging.

Natural does not have an official definition but is construed to mean the product does not contain artificial flavors, artificial colors or artificial preservatives.

Premium, Super Premium, Ultra Premium and Gourmet labeled foods are not required to contain higher quality ingredients, nor are they held to higher nutritional standards than are any other product.

With, such as "with real chicken," means that ingredient accounts for at least 3% of the food by weight, excluding water for processing.

Pet health experts see a definite trend towards home pet food preparation – whether completely from scratch or by adding to a base commercial diet. There are some basic diets now sold with the intention of having meat or eggs added to balance them. Many cats enjoy a bit of yogurt (if they aren't lactose-intolerant) or ground turkey added to their kibble.

When adding raw vegetables to a meal, throwing the greens into a food processor to break down the cellulose (the cell wall of green plants) can help your pet absorb the nutrients, but "wash them first!" And avoid onions, raisins, grapes, avocado and macadamia nuts, all of which can be toxic to your pets (see common poisons page 213).

With the raw food market continuing to expand as well as the arrival of packaged fresh frozen food (which does not require preservatives), it appears people are understanding the benefits and are getting back to basics for the health of their cats and dogs.

Regardless of your choice, educate yourself on feline and canine nutrition, practice proper hygiene and pay attention to how your pet responds to his food. Allergic reactions can present themselves as upset stomachs (vomiting and/or diarrhea), gas or belching, itchy skin or odorous infections, bald patches, constant paw or tail chewing, low energy to lethargy, hyperactivity, pale gums, bright red gums, rapid heart rate or breathing as well as anything that is not right with your pet. Tune in to notice any changes in your furry kid, and then take action by discussing with your Veterinarian or pet nutritionist. Advancements continue and there are new tests on the market that are less invasive and don't require your pet to be injected with allergens. Some tests screen for an elevation in antibodies. This could alert your Veterinarian early – when your cat's body is just starting to react or become sensitive. A saliva analysis streamlines the necessity of doing lengthy food trials (where one ingredient at a time is eliminated from your pet's diet) and may help get your furry companion on the path to a diet better suited for her.

Supplements:

Kittens, cats in the prime in the prime of their lives, and even our senior four-legged friends can benefit from supplements! Most pets just do not get proper vitamins, minerals and antioxidants in their diet, even when fed top-of-the-line food, so supplements can fill the gap. Commercial cat food sometimes contains by-products and useless fillers that can be toxic. Food with such ingredients can create unstable oxygen molecules - known as free radicals – which have been shown to cause a wide range of health problems including allergies, skin & coat problems, arthritis, tumors, cancer, cataracts, strokes and heart disease. Free radicals beat up the cells in our cat's bodies continuously throughout each day until they weaken the cells. Antioxidants are like super heroes dissolving these free radicals and protecting our pets. Another type of Supplement gaining popularity is Adaptogens. Adaptogens work with the body to read, repair and restore body system balance. Work with an pet herbal expert or holistic practitioner to choose the proper supplements for your pets and their particular needs.

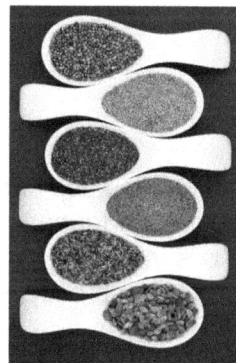

Once on supplements, you may not notice any outward change if your pet appears healthy, but know that a quality supplement is working inside your cat's body helping to keep the cells strong and healthy.

Consult with a knowledgeable Veterinarian or pet nutritionist to determine your cat's individual dietary needs. Some may benefit from a multi, whereas others will need specific vitamins, minerals or herbal remedies (see page 109 on Homeopathy).

Feeding The Instinctual Way:

Recently, the American Association of Feline Practitioners released a consensus statement that you should be reviewing how you are feeding your cat. They identified normal feeding behaviors in cats including noting that cats are meat eaters, carnivores, and that many domestic cats still possess a strong hunting instinct. Additionally, cats are solitary hunters who comsume small prey and will often prefer to eat alone and multiple times throughout the day. To engage these normal feline feeding behaviors, such as hunting and foraging, and eating frequent small meals in a solitary manner, look at options beyond the typical single bowl feeding approach. There are "No Bowl" feeding tools available that nurture and encourage your cat to fulfil it's natural instinct and hunt for smaller meals throughout the day. Their are an increasing number of feeding options like puzzle feeders and hunting solutions and it is becoming better understood that our cats physical, mental and instinctual health benefit from these feeding enrichment approaches.

6) Exercise & Stretching, Socialization & Basic Manners

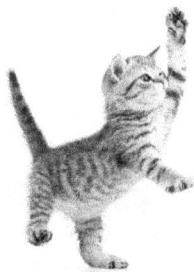

Exercise entertains your cat and keeps muscles toned, joints limber and weight under control. Cats may need to be tricked into exercising. Give your bundle of fur plenty of toys, perches and scratching posts, and play with her often. Make it fun! If your cat is alone during the day, consider getting her a feline friend to play and exercise with (see page 32 on Multiple Households).

Physical activity and fresh air do a feline body good…keeping your cat's body and mind sharp, but that fresh air is best consumed through a screened porch or catio. Even as your cat gets older, continue to keep her moving at a pace determined by your Veterinarian as boredom is the playground for bad habits and destructive behaviors like tearing this up, using inappropriate places to relieve herself and other unacceptable behaviors. Cats are natural hunters and need to keep busy. If you don't provide entertainment, they will find something to do!

Exercise ideas:

Swirl a feather toy, keep kitty active with puzzle games or get her a feline best friend to chase about the house.

Exercise may benefit your cat by:
- Lowering risks of arthritis, diabetes and other health related issues
- Keeping joints and ligaments limber and preventing muscle strains
- Delaying the loss of bone density
- Preventing muscles from atrophying
- Limiting weight gain
- Stimulating the brain

Stretching

Following exercise, stretch your feline friend – slowly and gently to decrease pain, improve mobility and increase his range of motion preventing future injuries. Stretching can improve the longevity and wellness of any feline.

This topic is a full volume on its own but areas to concentrate include the hips, shoulders and back. Done slowly and gently, most pets tolerate them well, however, if you feel uncertain, ask your Veterinarian, animal massage therapist or pet specific chiropractor to show you how.

Have your cat lying on her side if she prefers, except for the chest, stretch when she's on her back, belly up! Some animals feel vulnerable in this position, so don't force her on her back if that is the case as you will negate the effects by creating stress. If your cat shows any sign of pain during stretching, stop what you are doing and make a veterinary appointment ASAP.

- Chest muscles endure a great deal of strain. To stretch this area your goal is to carefully and gently pull the muscles away from center. With your cat on her back (if she is agreeable to this), grasp both front legs near the wrists and gently open them out to the side. Hold for 5 seconds, release and repeat. Feel free to relax her further with circular massage strokes to her chest or belly while in this position.

- Shoulder flexors create smooth movement in your cat's front legs. It is best if your cat will stand. Hold her front leg above the elbow while placing your other hand underneath the elbow, stabilizing it. Gently stretch her leg forward as if doing a "high five." At the point of resistance, hold the position 15 - 30 seconds and repeat 2 - 3 times for each front leg.

Not only does this stretch improve the integrity of the shoulders, wrists and elbows, but it can also increase breathing capacity by loosening chest muscles allowing for lung expansion.

- Hip Flexors are the muscles that allow your cat to move her legs and hips while walking or running. Best with your pet standing, hold her back leg above the knee, and gently stretch it straight back behind your cat's body. When you reach a point of resistance, where you'd actually be pulling the leg, stop and hold the position 15 - 30 seconds. Repeat 2 - 3 times with each back leg.

This stretch can increase flexibility in your cat's hips and spine while strengthening the lower back, hip and leg muscles. It may also lessen arthritis pain.

- Back stretching can be fun as it necessitates the use of treats! With your cat standing and you behind him or to one side, slowly move the treat from her nose towards her tail, encouraging your cat to follow with her eyes, only turning her head bending her body into a "C" shape. Make her hold the position for a count of 15 - 30 seconds, then repeat the exercise making the cat twist in the opposite direction. Do 2 - 3 stretches on each side. A good rub at the base of the tail, between the hip bones and up the spine feels especially good after this stretch. This helps increase the flow of spinal fluid and aids in the mobility of both your cat's hips and back.

Socializing:

Socializing goes hand-in-claw with obedience training. A well-socialized cat is friendly around other animals and people, is a welcome visitor to parks, pet-friendly locales and is an agreeable member of the family. She is less apt to get into a fight with other animals out of fear or bad manners.

Start early and slowly:

- Introduce your cat to family members and friends. Have them make her come and permit them to pet her in return for a treat or playtime with a feather on a string.
- Desensitize your cats to sounds around the house…vacuum cleaner, stereo, clapping hands, the doorbell, and…the neighboring dog's bark!

Basic Manners: Training

A well-behaved feline is less likely to escape into traffic or eat something she should not, so a trainer (and that can be YOU) should be part of your cat's Health & Safety Team! It is up to YOU to make sure that practice makes perfect.

Skills your kitty should excel at include:

- Accepting a friendly stranger
- Sitting politely for a petting
- Sitting nicely for grooming
- Come when called and stay in place, so as not to dash out an open door.

"STAY" COMMAND
"Stay" means your cat is not to move or leave the roo.

1) Once in the "Sit" position, use your flattened palm (like a "STOP" sign) in front of the kitty's face.

2) If she moves, tell her "no," take her back to "Sit" and start over.

3) Don't forget PRAISE for a job well done!

"LEAVE IT" COMMAND
'Leave It' means 'stop what you're doing' and can prevent your cat from consuming something she should not.. Use extra yummy treats to create more incentive.

1) Place an object (treat, toy, your slipper, etc.) in front of your cat while she is on a leash indoors so that you can control her movements.

2) As she moves towards it, say "Leave it."

3) If she stops in her tracks, say "Good Kitty," and treat her.

4) If not, pull back on her leash and try again.

Although cats are not taught obedience training to "stay" and not dash out the door and to "leave it" take to obedience training, it's a good idea to teach Fluffy to come when called. Using treats and a happy voice as a reward, teach kitty to respond to her name, the sound of an electric can opener or even a flickering light switch.

7) Educate Yourself and Don't Stop Learning for the Sake of Your Cat

There are so many opportunities these days to learn about animals - websites on every pet topic imaginable, webinars, YouTube videos, networks dedicated to animals, community college and classes at shelters, Agility for cats and kitty hotels & spas! Libraries offer lectures and book readings as well as shelves full of books on the subject. Radio and video programming (Internet, satellite and old-fashioned radio waves) bring a plethora of pet experts into your car or living room. Tune in and turn on to the vast array of information available about cats. Just do something, and keep on doing it for the sake of your four-legged best friend.

MASSAGE & YOUR PET

Massage may be the oldest and simplest form of medical care, and it may also be one of the most effective. Egyptian tombs display drawings of humans being massaged while Chinese writings (circa 2,700 BC) recommend "breathing, massage of skin and...exercises of hands and feet" as the appropriate treatment for many ailments. Julius Caesar was said to have been given a daily massage to treat neuralgia. In the 5th Century BC, Hippocrates, the father of Western Medicine wrote, "The physician must be experienced in many things, but assuredly in rubbing...for rubbing can bind a joint that is too loose, and loosen a joint that is too rigid." So why not use massage to help our four-legged friends too?

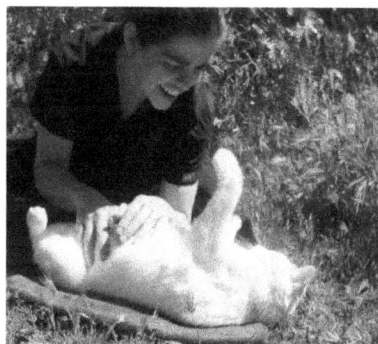

Photo Courtesy of Pam Holt.

Throughout history, massage has been used routinely on dogs and horses to aid and hasten recovery from injury, to provide relief from pain, and to calm and relax animals that live and work alongside humans. In the 21st Century, we are re-discovering the value of preventive care and recognizing the importance of viewing the body holistically. Our animal companions too are sharing the benefits as we implement natural and non-invasive modalities into their lives.

The power of massage comes from a focused touch. Basically, massage is touch with a purpose. According to Duke University Professor Dr. Saul Schanberg, "Touch is ten times stronger than verbal or emotional contact and is a key part to the survival of the animal species." In other words, touch is a biological need that affects almost every living creature!

Massage is the manipulation, methodical pressure, friction and kneading of the skin, muscle and soft tissues to achieve specific therapeutic results. Massage increases the flow of blood, nutrients and oxygen to all the tissues of the body which can accelerate the healing of an injury as well as the prevention of one by maintaining overall wellness. Injuries can be prevented by giving massage prior to heavy exercise and allowing your dog to warm-up and cool-down when participating in any type of sporting activity.

Massage for Injuries and Health

Massage therapy enhances every system of your pet's body – the immune, circulatory, endocrine, respiratory, nervous, digestive and lymphatic systems. Injury can be prevented if a pre-performance massage is given as muscles get warmed up with blood pumping through the tissues before activity begins.

Here are some additional benefits of massage:
- Stimulates the immune system which allows your cat to fight off infections.
- Increases the release of toxins from the body.
- Aids in the healing process.
- Lowers your cat's stress level and can have a calming effect on high-strung pets.
- Assists in training and competition as it creates focus.
- Increases the range and mobility of an animal's limbs thereby increasing their performance level.
- Relieves many of the discomforts of old age and degenerating conditions. Massage alleviates some of the pain and stiffness that comes with chronic arthritis and hip dysplasia.
- Creates a deeper bond between you and your cat while building confidence, trust and affection.

To *warm-up*, start with slow long continuous strokes (effleurage) from head to tail, down the outside and up the inside of limbs, gently increasing the pressure as you go. This will increase circulation, stretch the muscle fibers and warm the tissues. Have patience. Especially with kitties, it may take a while for them to begin to enjoy massage

Once you have warmed the muscles up, apply friction with your thumbs and fingers across the muscle fibers followed by the deeper petrissage. With your thumbs and fingers, gently knead and roll the skin improving oxygenation to the tissues. Begin lightly and increase pressure to release toxins and spasms from the muscles while bringing blood and nutrients to them. This is critical to their flexibility and movement for the competition ahead.

Conclude with more long strokes and gently stretch and flex your feline by extending her limbs while always maintaining support of them. End the massage with more effleurage to clear the muscles of her metabolic waste.

Finish up with lots and lots of long strokes. Gently compress to drain the muscles of lactic acid that can be painful if allowed to build up. Since the muscles have been exerted during the course of exercise, use a lighter touch during your post-performance massage. Make slower and slower strokes as you attempt to cool the body down. Finish off with a cool refreshing bowl of water to aid in the elimination of toxins.

Massage and stretching can be very beneficial for dogs with hip dysplasia, cruciate or back surgery, but of course every animal is different. Massage and proper rehabilitation of a post-surgical anterior cruciate rupture may help prevent the need for surgery in the non-surgical leg. Most dogs, within a year's time, end up tearing the non-surgical ACL due to additional stress placed on it during recovery of the first leg.

Who Should Massage Your Pet?

Find someone who is certified in animal-specific massage therapy so that they're familiar with the anatomy and physiology of your pet. Like with your Veterinarian, groomer or anyone you entrust your four-legged family member to, make sure there is a connection between the person and your pet. Make sure you are comfortable with the energy coming from them since the masseuse's energy will be transferred to your pet.

Do-It-Yourself Massage Techniques and Guidelines

NOTE: Never massage an animal that has a fever or is exhibiting signs of shock, heat stroke or distress. In these cases, get your pet to the vet! Massage is designed to increase circulation and could work against the body's natural defenses. Also if a pet has osteoporosis (fragile bones), massage could be too intense. Steer clear of areas that are bruised, blistered or show signs of a rash. For any of these conditions, talk with your Veterinarian.

1) Familiarize yourself with the basic techniques of massage:
   - **Effleurage** – Long gentle strokes in the direction of the fur using your whole flat palm and fingers.
   - **Finger Tip Pressure/Friction Massage** – Use two or three fingers or your thumbs across the muscle fibers following down the fur line in circular movements with a little shaking (but don't take your fingers off your cat's skin). Fast and invigorating, apply firm pressure but do not press deeply into muscle or tissue.
   - **TTouchesTM®** – Small circular movements of the fingers and hands all over the body making one and one-quarter circles (Visualize small clock faces and go from six o'clock all the way around past six and up to nine o'clock with your fingertips). Learn more at www.ttouch.com
   - **Acupressure Pointwork** – Press down gently and hold for five to thirty seconds in areas next to or between muscles, bones, vertebrae and around joints. Do not press on bony prominences or into the belly of the muscle. Exhale as you press and then inhale as you let up off the point.
   - **Petrissage** – Deeper massage consisting of gentle kneading, compressing, rolling and wringing of the skin, picking up and squeezing warm, relaxed muscles.
   - **Stretches** – Only after muscles have been warmed up, slowly stretch your pet's legs in their normal direction, never going past the point of resistance.
   - **Tapotement** – Gentle tapping to stimulate circulation.
   - **Closure** – Effleurage and then just passive touch by placing your hands for short periods of time on your pet's body without any pressure or movement.

2) Make sure your cat is ready! She shouldn't be hungry, but it is best if she hasn't eaten for at least an hour before receiving a massage. A walk or litterbox is a good idea before hand to let her empty her bladder and expend energy so that she will be more willing to relax.

3) Wash your hands and then rub them together to get your energy and circulation flowing.

4) Always ask the kitty for her permission before you begin. The response should be obvious, if you tune in, and you should always honor it.

5) A positive attitude is crucial! Your energy is going to be passed on to your cat, so never begin a massage if you are in a bad mood, stressed, tired or carrying negative energy of any type. Close your eyes, take a deep breath and exhale, sending your worries away while you too relax during this special time with your feline friend. Try to match the cadence of your breathing to your pet's respiration so that the two of you are more in tune.

6) Create a calm ambiance by finding a quiet space. Lay a sheet on the floor, dim the lights and play soothing music at a low volume to mask distracting noises.

7) Always keep both hands on your cat throughout the massage so that you maintain a constant connection, paying attention to any feedback she gives you.

8) Be conscious of trigger points which will feel like a knot in the center of a muscle. These spots are tender, so apply light pressure with your thumb until you feel the muscle release. Then use long strokes to drain the muscle of the lactic acid.

9) Make sure you massage both sides of your pet for balance.

10) After the massage, offer your pet fresh water to help flush out the toxins and lactic acid that you have moved around.

Other Disciplines that Aid Injuries and Promote Health in Pets

A combination of non-invasive modalities can be used after surgery and along with massage during the course of rehabilitation therapy.

Acupuncture: Using acupuncture needles can stimulate specific points on the body resulting in various physiological effects including increased blood flow, the release of endorphins (natural pain killers), the production of cortisol which acts as an anti-inflammatory, and an increase of white blood cells and antibodies which stimulate the immune system. Besides needle insertion, acupuncture encompasses the following techniques:

- Acupressure: Administration of pressure to specific points on the body to create an effect similar to needle insertion. This is great for harder to insert locations and pets who may not take to needles.
- Aquapuncture: Liquids (homepathics, diluted vitamins such as B12 and certain medications) are injected exerting an energetic change by pushing tissue out of their way.

- Moxibustion: Applying a heated herbal compound to needles prior to insertion. This can benefit older pets and those suffering from joint and muscular conditions.
- Laser: A needle-less treatment for patients that don't tolerate needle insertion – a cool laser stimulates acupressure points without burning the skin or hair. See more below.
- Electrostimulation or Estim: Coursing electric current into the body between needles that have been inserted into acupuncture points can relax spasming muscles and assist the body in reestablishing nervous system impulses when nerve damage has occurred, such as spinal cord damage from a ruptured disc.

Animal Communication: Humans who possess the gift of being able to really tune into our animals may help you find out why your pet is behaving a certain way, what may ail them or any other story they wish you would know. Communicators use various techniques to do telepathic reads (like a conversation), energy dowsing (to find blocks in energy pathways), chakra scans and flower essence reads (checking for emotional balance) along with other tools to help you better know what your pet can't tell you, or you can't understand. Discovering an area of discomfort in your pet through communication could help a medical practitioner zero in on a problem and hopefully come up with a solution.

Aromatherapy: Aromatherapy is the therapeutic inhalation often by the means of hydrosols or mists of pure essential oils to restore or enhance health and well-being. Essential oils come from various parts of aromatic plants -- the rind, flower, bark, root, resin or leaf -- that are released via steam distillation, cold expression or solvent extraction. They should not be confused with fragrance oils and potpourri, which can contain synthetic ingredients that can cause problems, such as headaches, agitation or allergic reactions. Never use essential oils directly on a cat, even when diluted. Don't try ANY on your feline best friend without working a professional highly trained in essentials oils for cats. Cats can have an adverse reaction to essential oils. Cat's livers lack the ability to metabolize and detoxify many of these substances, so know which essential oils are safe specifically for cats. Remember that a cat's sense of smell is much more sensitive than ours, so whatever you are using in their environment, will impact them.

Chiropractic: Chiropractic manipulations or adjustments aid joints and help relax muscles by restoring misaligned vertebrae to their proper position in your cat's spinal cord. The underlying philosophy is that disease results from a disruption of nerve function, primarily caused by displaced vertebrae. When a veterinary chiropractic procedure is done, the goal is to re-align the spine relieving pressure on nerves. Followed by massage, chiropractic can be very effective.

Veterinary Orthopedic Manipulation (VOM): Not quite chiropractic, but a close cousin, Veterinary Orthopedic Manipulation (VOM) was developed by a veterinary neurologist (Dr. William Inman) who discontinued his surgical practice after seeing the outstanding benefits of this technology. VOM is a healing technique focused on returning an animal's nervous system to a healthy state. This is done with a hand held device called an Activator which reduces subluxations – misalignments of the bones. Out of place discs and joints slightly out of their socket are prime contenders for this treatment, and problems may be found with this method months prior to them showing up on x-rays. Most pets tolerate the light pressure and if repeated, the process actually releases endorphins causing the animal to relax. When fired down the spine, the Activator can open up blockages in the nerve bundles on either side aiding the various internal organs as well.

Hydrotherapy/Underwater Treadmill: The buoyancy of water allows exercise with less stress to the joints and can have cardiovascular benefits. The warmth of the water helps increase circulation, relax muscles and allows for greater flexibility and range of motion. Hydrotherapy can also decrease inflammation and swelling and reduce pain levels.

Hyperbaric Oxygen Therapy (HBOT): Hyperbaric comes from the Greek word "hyper" meaning "more" and "baric" relating to pressure. A hyperbaric oxygen chamber increases the pressure allowing a patient's body to absorb much larger quantities of oxygen than it would if it was not under pressure. When oxygen is inhaled at normal atmospheric pressure, it is transported on hemoglobin in the red blood cells. Under pressure, however, oxygen dissolves in the plasma, cerebrospinal fluid in the brain and spinal cord, lymph and other body fluids making it more easily delivered to the tissues, including those with poor blood supply.

Oxygen deprivation due to poor circulation, injury, surgery and other causes can hinder healing and impair function, which is why HBOT benefits so many diverse conditions including:

- Snakebites and Traumatic Injuries such as crushing, swelling & major vessel tears
- Pressure Sores & Chronic Wounds
- Carbon Monoxide Poisoning
- Severe Anemia
- Severe Gastrointestinal Illness
- Bone Infections
- Stroke

One of the most dramatic examples of oxygen deprivation would be during a stroke. A blockage or bleeding in the brain's blood vessels disrupts the flow of oxygen as well as nutrient-rich blood. Cells in the affected area die or are damaged, but when these areas are infused with massive amounts of oxygen during a hyperbaric oxygen treatment, damaged brain cells may literally wake up.

LLLT/Cold Laser/Therapeutic Laser: Low-Level Laser Therapy, Low Level Light Therapy or "cold laser" is a non-thermal light energy used to stimulate healing, reduce inflammation and provide pain relief. Benefits may include stimulation of both cartilage and collagen and can assist dogs suffering from arthritis, tendonitis, muscle spasm and various wounds.

Nutrition: Proper nutrients are critical to create a healthy immune system and good body condition. Proper nutrition can add several years to your cat's life and delay the need for medication for chronic diseases such as osteoarthritis. You may want to consider supplements depending on the nutrition path that you've chosen for your pets as no one diet is perfect for every cat. Speak with a professional to customize what may help your animal thrive. See pages 12 - 17 for more nutrition information.

Holistic Approach: Increasingly, cat parents are considering alternative treatments for their pets for a variety of reasons. A holistic approach is one that factors in the entire body and being of the pet – it looks at the big picture and sees how everything is working together to create a whole and healthy animal. Rather than fixing a problem, it seeks the root causes addressing it in a "gentle healing" method for long-term results. More and more Veterinarians and other professionals are incorporating holistic and homeopathic treatments and approaches into western medicine. If this is something that resonates with you, seek out a specialized professional in that area and discuss the options and expectations.

Knowledge is power and more and more is discovered each year in our quest to help cats live longer, happier, healthier lives. Take advantage of the seminars and workshops, webinars, websites, good old fashioned books and the expertise of professionals who live to help pets thrive. Refer to the charts and forms in the back of this book and be proactive by filling them out and seeking out the information you don't currently possess. You are your pet's advocate and protector.

Notes: _____

_____

_____

_____

_____

_____

_____

_____

_____

_____

CBD for your Cats

CBD has been gaining in popularity in the pet world as way to address a variety of wide ranging health and wellness conditions. Though research on it and the Endocannabinoid System (ECS) are still in what would deemed the early stages, compared to other body systems, there is much to be encouraged by from what has been researched, as well as a multitude of anecdotal evidence.

So What is CBD?
CBD is an acronym for Cannabidiol (Can-a-bid-i-ol), a naturally occurring class of molecules called cannabinoids abundant in the plant genus Cannabis Sativa L. CBD makes up close to 40% of the plant and is just one of over 100 cannabinoids presently identified in cannabis sativa. CBD interacts with an animal's naturally occurring endocannabinoid system, and is non-psychoactive because there is little to no THC (tetrahydrocannabinol). In brief, CBD or PCR (Phyto Cannabinoid Rich) sativa plants having low levels of THC are referred to as Hemp and Marijuana plants are those with high levels of THC.

A bit more about Hemp vs. Marijuana

Hemp and marijuana are related, but the differences can be night and day.

- First off, the plants look different. One of the oldest domestic crops grown, tall, sturdy hemp plants were farmed by early civilizations for food, oil, shelter and textiles. Similar to bamboo, shoots can grow 15 feet high. Marijuana plants however, tend to grow as low and bushy.
- As far as cultivation, hemp is grown for its stalks and seeds and marijuana for its leaves and flowers.
- The elevated levels of THC in marijuana are responsible for its signature "high," while hemp has very little THC. A study done by a private laboratory in Denver (Charas Scientific) found that recreational marijuana contains up to 30% THC while the hemp used to create products for pets and people contains a maximum legal amount of .03%. Some companies even go through a costly process to remove all traces of THC in hemp products to improve safety.
- Both hemp and marijuana contain CBD, but the hemp plant produces more, making it the preferred choice to battle anxiety, chronic pain, epilepsy and other ailments. Since CBD does not cause a "high," it is considered a holistic treatment, not a pharmaceutical one.

So keep in mind that CBD and Marijuana are definitely not the same and only one – CBD – is safe for pets. Never ever share edibles, THC or any human-specific cannabis products with your cat! "The number-one animal ER issue in states in which medical and/or recreational marijuana is legal is marijuana intoxication," says Dr. Robin Downing, DVM and a pain medicine veterinary specialist

Are all CBD oils created equal?

No. Many CBD oils on the market are NOT naturally occurring NOR are they truly full spectrum CBD. Most undergo a form of chemical synthesis that requires lab manipulation - compounds are taken out during the extraction process and synthesized ones added in. In order to be considered a truly full spectrum CBD oil (which is what you want for your pet), it should contain naturally occurring (Phyto-Cannabinoid Rich) therapeutic parts of the plant. You need to know how the plants were grown and how the compounds were extracted in order to get the best quality CBD oil for your pet!

The hemp plant is considered a hyper-accumulator which means it readily absorbs anything in the soil. So it is even important to know what kinds of soil, and what pest control methods were used in the growth of the plants.

How does it work?

Dogs, cat, humans, all invertebrates (except insects) have an endocannabinoid system that helps maintain the physiological, neurological and immunological systems of the body -- it modulates our emotions, response to pain and other sensations. If there is a deficiency anywhere, multiple receptors can use CBD oil to help the body get into balance or achieve homeostasis. We still have much to learn yet findings are already showing the symbiotic relationship between the Endocannabinoid system in our bodies and CBD.

Awonderful benefit of how CBD interacts with the body's own endocannabinoid system is known as the entourage effect. This is when the many components within the cannabis plant interact with the body to produce a stronger influence than any one of those components alone. When we combine multiple compounds, we don't end up with the sum of each part but exponentially increase their effects.

How much CBD oil should I give my cat?

CBD interacts with your pet's endocannabinoid system, which means their reaction is dependent on their tolerance as well as immunity. In other words, every pet is a bit different. Surprisingly, CBD dosage is not dependent exclusively on weight, however it can be a guideline. "Start low and go slow" until you achieve the results you are seeking for your pet is the mantra. Recommending dosage is 0.05 mg per lbs. twice daily slowly increasing to to 0.25 mg per lbs. twice daily.

For cats, Dr. Celeste Yarnall suggested, "Put one drop in the palm of your hand...mix it with a little water or wild-caught organic sardine oil. Many cats really love having their gums massaged."

While there is more to learn about CBD (AKA – PCR Hemp Oil), it is showing to be a multi-modality aid for pain, nausea, anxiety and a number of other ailments without causing the organ and tissue damage NSAIDs (anti-inflammatory meds), anti-convulsants and other pharmaceuticals can cause.

READING YOUR CAT'S BODY LANGUAGE

On a daily basis, study your pet and learn to communicate with him, gaining his trust and paying close attention to what he is trying to say through Body Language. When any animal is upset or not feeling well, even your own best friend, they might be grumpy and could nip, so it's important to stay alert to changes in their ears, eyes, tail, vocalization and muscle tension. Any animal (just like a human) may be in a good mood one moment and then do a 180, so stay alert to even the slightest changes.

The following is a general guideline but knowing your own pet's personality is the best measure. Additional drawings are in the Resource Section of this book to get you better acquainted as to what the various behaviors look like.

	Happy Cat	Sour Puss	Scaredy Cat	Sick Cat
Ears	Flat	Flat & Pressed Back Against Head	Pulled Back Against Head	To The Sides Or Any Abnormal Position
Eyes	Open & Bright	Pupils Narrow	Wide Open	Half Crossed
Hackles (Fur on the neck & back)	Relaxed & Smooth Fur	Fluffed Up	Fluffed Up	Could Go Either Way
Tails	Relaxed or upright especially if the tip of the tail is curled can mean "howdy". May lower front legs with butt in the air waggin tail with a "play bow".	Swishing with hair bristled or straight up like a bottle brush.	Tucked between legs or he'll bow with hair standing straight up.	Tucked Between Legs
Whiskers	Straight To The Side	Pulled Back Against Face	Forward Or Back	Pulled Forward Or Any Abnormal Position
Sounds	Gentle purring and meows.	Hissing or spitting, cats even chatter when frustrated.	Frightened cry to growing or hissing.	Cats may purr when comforted.
Rubbing Behavior	When cats rub against you or scratch objects they are leaving their scent saying you are their property; a sign of endearment			

Proper Handling

For a cat to enjoy (or even tolerate) being picked up, she must feel secure and trust you completely. Her body must always be supported, and she will show displeasure if you allow her hind legs to dangle. With kittens, care must be taken not to bruise their tiny rib cage by grabbing hold too tightly.

Knowing how to properly "scruff" a cat can be helpful in getting her into a carrier for a trip to the Veterinarian or to restrain her while administering first-aid. Scruffing is similar to the way a mother cat carries her young and is a good way to discourage undesirable behavior if done properly. When scruffed, most cats go still. If yours does not, use a towel to control her (see below).

To Scruff:

Photo Courtesy of Sunny-dog Ink.

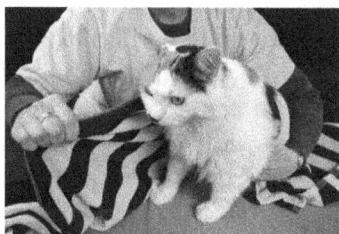

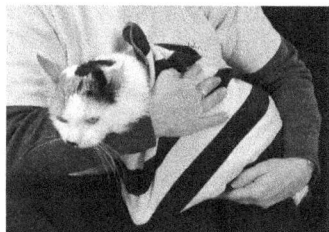

- Place your hand at the base of the cat's head below the ears and above the shoulders and grab the loose skin pulling up slightly. The skin should pull with little resistance. Long-haired cats may seem harder to scruff due to the thick layer of hair.
- Supporting kitty's hind legs, carefully lift and quickly carry her where you need her to go (crate, table top).
- Otherwise, gently push the kitty towards the floor or other surface until her muscles relax if you're scruffing to discipline or control the cat.
- Making a "hissing" sound before you say "no" to an unruly feline may remind her of mom's reprimands.
- If your cat is still not cooperating, wrap a towel around her covering all four legs, as if swaddling a baby. It may calm her but if not, the towel should lessen her scratches.
- Always be gentle and reassure your cat with soothing words and a comforting pet when you are done. Then give her some space.

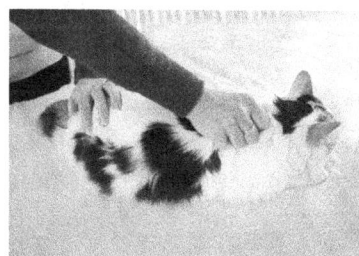

Photos Courtesy of Sunny-dog Ink.

Wrap Your Cat In a Towel To Restrain Her   Kitty Purrito - Restraining Your Cat To Perform First Aid

To learn more about muzzling and restraining for at-home procedures, turn to page 98 in the Pet First-Aid section of this book.

INTRODUCTIONS

Introducing Your Cat to a New Feline Family Member:

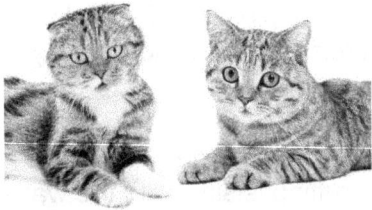

It is likely your cat will react to a newcomer by distancing herself. She may hide refusing to acknowledge the new cat, or she may act up in an attempt to persuade the new feline to retreat.

To make the introduction go smoothly:

- Put your new cat in a spare room with the door closed for the first few days allowing both kitties a chance to adjust to each other's scents (by sniffing under doors) without hurting each other.
- Give each of them a towel or blanket that the other cat has laid on to familiarize them with each other's scent.
- If your cats exhibit personality conflicts, you can reduce tension by making sure each cat has enough personal space and personal possessions to fulfill her needs.
- To avoid territory conflicts, place litter boxes in several locations throughout your home.

Introducing Cats and Dogs

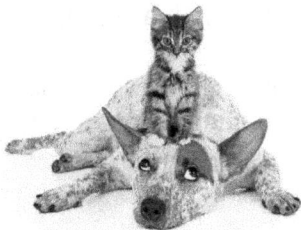

Some do fine. Some cannot live safely together. The first rule is proceed cautiously during introductions having at least two people present, one ready to intervene with each animal if need be.

Keep the dog on a loose lead and observe his body language at all times. The other person should pay attention to the cat's reactions. Do not push the animals together. If the cat is not raising her hackles (the fur on her back) or hissing, allow her to move freely around the room. If the dog is not acting aggressively, praise him as he allows the cat to move around, even sniffing the dog if she wishes. Dogs with strong prey instincts will become focused, staring, stiffening, whining and/or barking. If these behaviors are present or if the dog lunges, calmly put the cat in another room with a tall baby gate while one person distracts the dog playing with a toy.

When set up with the cat in another room with all her supplies and a tall and sturdy baby gate installed in the door, allow the dog periodic loose leash visits to see the cat on the other side of the gate. Once the cat no longer creates such a rise in the dog, sit comfortably on the floor on the dog's side of the gate and reach through, petting the cat and feeding her treats on her side while you do the same with the dog.

Your goal is to lessen your dog's interest in your feline companion, but in some cases, instinct is strong and the two may never be left safely alone. If introductions are not going well, seek a professional behaviorist. In the worst circumstances, a dog can quickly injure or kill a cat and cats can inflict devastating eye injuries on dogs. Calm, patient baby steps are the best route to getting these two species comfortable around each other.

Introducing your Cat to Your New Baby

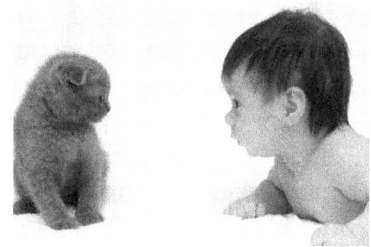

Animals, like their two-legged counterparts, can cope with big changes in their lives if we take the time to help them through. A new human brother or sister joining the family is an exciting time for all but can be stressful with added noise, stressed out parents and possibly less time for belly rubs and ear scratches. Doing your homework and properlypreparing your cat can make for a smooth transition. Don't wait for the day your newborn comes home to start telling your pet how to behave! You are setting him up for disaster if you do so and that is completely unfair.

If you are pregnant, you have probably heard of toxoplasmosis since it can cause serious birth defects. Do not be alarmed or jump to conclusions feeling you need to give away your cat. The disease is quite rare in the United States and can be easily avoided. Ask your obstetrician to perform a simple blood test to determine if you are immune. If not, avoid handling or eating raw or uncooked meat, keep your cat indoors and away from wildlife (especially birds and mice) and have someone else clean out the litter box for duration of your pregnancy. If you are a gardener, always wear gloves as neighborhood cats may "go" in your garden.

If you haven't already, start looking at your cat like you are her parent too. Is she lacking manners and socialization that could prove dangerous around a baby or even pregnant you? Start now correcting any behaviors you've, up to now, over looked. Gently tug, bump and squeeze her paws a little at a time to acclimate her as to how the baby might touch her. If she responds well, praise, praise, praise! If she is uncomfortable, she needs to learn to walk away to her own space and not bite or hiss. If your cat won't let you get away with this "tougher" handling, he or she certainly won't let the baby.

A big change for your pet with the baby's arrival will be the amount of time you get to devote to her each day. Do not ignore her, but start preparing her by varying meal and walk times and quality versus quantity of special time together. Make sure she has a special space to retreat to and plenty of toys to keep her busy when you can't. Begin weaning your cat off cat toys that in any way resemble baby toys. Find play things for Fluffy that are uniquely different so that there won't be confusion later on with your cat thinking the baby has her toy!

Do let your cat explore the nursery as you set it up and accustom kitty to the movements of an empty stroller. Even practice with a doll in the stroller going for walks together. If you have friends with babies, having them visit and letting your cat meet their babies under supervision can be a great help. Always let the cat go slowly to the baby. Do not push a baby into an animal's face! Practice helps smooth the way and helps your cat learn what to expect.

Help your kitty learn to adjust to the new sounds and smells. Let them sniff baby powders and oils on your hands, baby wipes and even the smell of pureed carrots long before your baby comes home.

While you are in the hospital, a great trick is to send home a blanket or clothing the baby has slept on or worn. Then let your cat get familiar with the scent before the baby's homecoming.

When the moment arrives for introductions, come in first without the baby so your cat can give you their proper greeting and you'll have free hands to return their affection. Once the initial hellos have been accomplished, have another family member bring in the baby and slowly let your cat meet his new "brother or sister." Watch body language but remember…pets pick up your vibes, so stay calm but alert. Take care with your voice. "Baby talk" to your baby could be mistaken for the sounds you use for your cat and might sound like an invitation for her to play or interact with the baby.

Although baby will be foremost on your mind, try to give your cat as much one-on-one time as possible. Having spent time teaching her down/stay commands and playing quietly with toys in her special space will really pay off now.

No matter how well things are going, NEVER EVER leave your baby and cat alone together… An animal's natural instincts could be triggered by a crying or cooing infant.

Remember too, that you will be bringing all types of new things into the house and many may drop and land on the floor. Pay due diligence to keep your cat safe from pins, buttons and anything that your cat could swallow or could cause her harm.

A few special notes about our feline friends: remember, they especially do not like a change to their routine or lifestyle. Try to keep their routine as normal as possible, even if you have a pet sitter come in to brush, feed and create playtime. Doing many of the things mentioned previously (playing recordings of a baby crying, letting your cat explore the nursery and sniff items the baby has worn) work well to smooth the transition for your cat as well.

It is an old wives' tale about cats smothering babies or sucking the breath out of them. A cat should never lose her home when a human comes in to the world. Plan ahead for a happy lifetime together.

Show patience and love, always supervise and stay alert to your cat's and your baby's changing attitudes so you can quickly make any corrections along the way. Think about little things like keeping your cats well-groomed and practice training to be sure they continue to mind their manners. If things aren't going well, don't delay. Seek the immediate help of a professional behaviorist or trainer to nip it in the bud. With love, patience and effort, you can enjoy watching your child and cat becoming loyal companions and playmates.

On a final note, keep in mind the amazing ways your cat might HELP with your baby:

- Baby Monitor: Cats and their amazing ears will be on high alert.

- Entertainment: Giggles and smiles will ensue when baby watches kitty chase her tail.

- Immune Booster: Studies have shown that the exposure to germs from cats challenges a child's immune system leading to fewer respiratory illnesses and ear infections as well as a decreased risk for asthma and allergies later in life.

- Clean-up: Make sure what drops is feline safe and that they do not take food from the child.

- Unconditional Love: There's nothing a child needs in never-ending supply more than love and your happy, well-mannered cat is a perfect source of unwavering devotion.

Be sure to read about "Zooeyia" on page 5 to understand more fully the benefits our four-legged friends can have on your child and on you.

Introducing your Cat to Visitors/Strangers

Having your cat meet family and friends can be an exciting and rewarding time. Particularly if the people are not cat savvy, talk to them ahead about what to expect and what you'd prefer they do and don't do when Fluffy greets them. Sudden movements, hand clapping and foot stomping can scare or put your cat on guard. Also beware that although some people may say, "I love animals," they could be referring to the older fluffy Siamese they had as a child and not your rambunctious two-year old Bengal cat, so give them a heads-up as to your cat's personality so that everyone starts off on the same page. Having a brief phone conversation with visitors prior to their ringing the bell will help keep the peace. Remind them to pull closed screen doors and latch any gates, not to feed your pets unless you provide a treat and to watch what they bring into your home (medication in purses, cigarettes and lighters).

As the person enters, have your cat stay away from the door and let them know when it's okay to nose over. After your cat has had a good sniff, tell the person to offer the back of their hand for an additional nose-over and then to gently extend their fingers under the cat's chin for a gentle scratching or petting. Children in particular must learn not to pat a cat on the head which looks like a slap or hit to the animal and can immediately make him defensive.

Pet Friendly Kid Tips

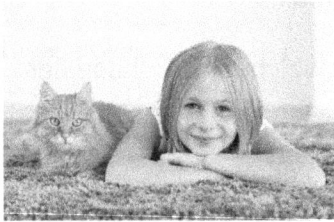

To safely share our lives with our four-legged friends,
there are **tips every human should follow,**
no matter their number of years on the planet:

Never, ever leave a child alone with a pet!!!

NEVER

- Tease cats by pulling their ears or tails.
- Throw things at them or chase them.
- Touch or play with a kittyl while she is eating or sleeping.
- Steal toys or bones.
- Run or scream if an animal comes near you and never run towards him.
- Stare into an cat's eyes.
- Do not pat kitty on the head. This looks like you are going to hit her. Instead, let her sniff the back of your hand (after you have asked permission to pet the cat) and if the cat seems agreeable, extend your fingers and slowly beginning to scratch under her chin and neck.

ALWAYS

- Act kindly and gently towards animals.
- Ask if it is okay before you pet someone else's cat.
- Stand still like a tree if an animal comes near you, and allow her to sniff you first. Then scratch under her chin if he seems agreeable, but never raise your hand above her head which looks like a slap.
- Tell an adult if you see a stray or injured animal.

Animals can magically put a smile on any human face. For all they do for us, we must learn to treat them with compassion and learn to speak their language, allowing them their own space and time.

BASIC CAT CARE

Seven "Purrfectly GOOD TO KNOW" Rules to Help YOU Help YOUR Cat

1) Give your kitty a weekly *Head-to-Tail Check-up* monitoring respiration, pulse, capillary refill time and feeling for lumps & bumps, fleas, ticks, foxtails, etc. Finding a lump early and getting it checked could save your pet's life. Observe your cat's normal habits (notice how much she drinks, eats, urinates & defecates); notice her stance and how she sits. If you know what's normal for your cat, you can quickly notice something that is not and alert your Veterinarian. (See page 208)

2) Spay or Neuter your cat and take him to the Veterinarian for *annual check-ups*, including wellness or geriatric testing once your cat reaches age 7. Keep good records on your cat's health, licensing and care issues, and learn where your closest animal emergency center is in case your vet is closed when you need her.

3) Although indoor cat's do not always wear collars, have an *ID tag* on your cat's collar for when she does, and get her microchipped so she can find her way home should she ever become separated from you. Keep these identifiers up-to-date and make sure tags are legible as the lettering tends to wear off over time.

4) *Socialize & Obedience Train & Exercise your cat*. Socialize your cat and teach her a few rules. A cat who knows her manners is less likely to get into less likely to get into trouble and a well-socialized pet will become a more-welcomed member of the family. *Always keep you cat indoors or in an enclosed patio so that you can keep her safe from traffic or in a fenced yard* so that you can keep her safe from traffic, other animals, pesticides that might be on your neighbor's lawn, poisons in garbage cans and more. Many well-meaning owners expose their cats to needless dangers by allowing their animals to run loose. Since we've domesticated our dogs and cats, changed their landscape and created motor cars and super highways, we have an obligation to restrict our pets' boundaries to keep them out of harm's way. How often have you seen an animal hit by a car on a street near you? You certainly don't want your four-legged friend to suffer this fate. Additionally, stray pets are often killed by other animals, poisoned, contract disease or are sold to labs for experimentation. Regardless of the size of land you inhabit, it is imperative that you create a big enough world at home for your animals to explore and thrive in.

Exercise your cat. Keep your kitty's body and mind stimulated for a long, happy and healthy life. Boredom is the playground for bad habits and destructive behaviors.Physical and mental activity does a feline body good, but so does but so does time spent with you!

5) Feed a *high quality, age-appropriate food* (kitten food for kitties, senior food for older cats, light food for overweight pets) and read those labels so that you know what you're really feeding your best friend. Also give supplements for long-term nutritional therapy which protect your pet from the inside out & provide nutrients commercial food may lack. Check with your Veterinarian or pet nutritionist to find out what is advised.

6) Finally, please make sure you keep your cat's body & mind stimulated with plenty of *exercise, play time and time spent with YOU.*

7. *Know Cat Safety & Learn Cat First Aid & CPCR* (see Section Two)…It could save a life! Also put together a *Cat First-Aid Kit* (page 99) so that you'll have the tools to do the job.

Weekly Head-to-Tail Check-up (also see page 208)

Really get to know your cat and you'll more quickly identify something 'not quite right!' Getting your cat used to your touch not only can help you find a small problem before it becomes a nightmare, but will also make your cat's Health & Safety Team happier since they (your Veterinarian, groomer and pet sitter) will find her much easier to handle. Keep a record of your observations on the diagram located in the resource section of this book entitled "Head-To-Tail". (See pages 208)

Look & feel your cat over from head-to-tail:

- Check ears for foul odor or redness.
- Make sure eyes look clear, pupils are equally dilated and there's no excessive tearing.
- Kitty breath should not be offensive; smelling sweet or like nail polish remover could signal kidney problems.
- Feel for lumps and bumps - catching a tumor early could save a life.
- If your cat's skin is flaky or her coat is dull, bathe, brush and add Omega 3s to her diet.
- Remove parasites, burrs or foxtails.
- Check paw pads for cracks and make sure nails are trimmed short.
- Keep private areas clean.

Notice changes in your cat's behavior or routine. If your cat is requiring you to perform these tasks more or less frequently he may need a check-up:

- Refilling water bowls
- Amount of food being consumed
- How often litter needs to be changed
- Soiled spots in the house

Get familiar with what your cat looks like when she sits, stands and walks.
"Yes" to any of these questions means it's time for a visit to your Veterinarian:

- Is her posture unusual?
- Is it more difficult for my cat to get up or lie down or does she moan when doing so?
- Is she leaning to one side or favoring a limb?
- Is she less active?

Notes:

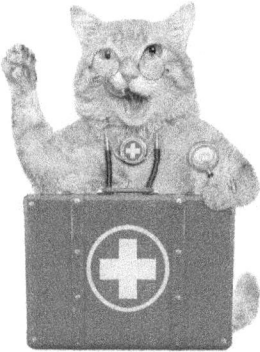

Check	Your Cat Is Good To Go	How You Can Help	Your Cat Needs To Go To The Veterinarian
Ears	Pink and Smell Good	Wax debris - clean with ear wash	Foul odor, redness or ear mites which look like coffee grounds
Eyes	Bright & clear, pupils are equally dilated & responsive; no excessive tearing	Excessive Tearing - Flush with saline solution or eye wash	Cloudiness to eyes; one pupil larger than the other; excessive tearing not alleviated by saline solution or eye wash; squinting or pawing at eye.
Nose	Shiny & Moist		Dry & cracked excessively dripping; mucus discharge; sneezing; open wound.
Mouth	Clean white teeth with no bad odor; scissor bite from teeth meeting properly; pink moist gums with CRTs less than 2 seconds	Brush daily with pet specific toothpaste. Keep pet well hydrated.	Foul odor, tartar build up; redness obvious absess or loose teeth; uneven bite; brightened, blue, pale or white; dry or tacky gums.
Skin & Coat	Shiny, no lumps, or bumps or flakes; healthy pink; no hair loss.	Bathe, brush regularly & add Omega 3s to your dog's diet.	Lumps, bumps, scabs, open sores; bald spots or extreme hair loss.
Legs & Paws	When walking, gait is smooth & even. No cuts to pads; nails short; cat stands and moves well with no tenderness. Did you know cats have 5 toes on the front paws and 4 on the back? Those with more are referred to as polydactyl.	Clean any pads wounds. Don't let them walk on hot or extremely cold surfaces; trim nails ; exercise.	Open wounds; limping; unsteadiness; difficulty walking;, getting up or lying down; dragging a limb.
Chest & Abdomen	Pink skin, no lumps, bumps or tender areas.; you can feel ribs but not see them and chest is lower than the tummy	*Keep your pet at a healthy weight.*	*Any lumps or tenderness; need to lose excessive weight.*
Heart	Steady even rythm. 90-220 Beats Pet Minute for small dogs and cats	Get regular veterinary check ups and appropriate exercise.	Murmur or uneven heart beats (arrhythmia); faster or slower rate of BPM than normal.

Check	Your Cat Is Good To Go	How You Can Help	Your Cat Needs To Go To The Veterinarian
Lungs	Clear inhalation and exhalation. 20 - 40 Beats Pet Minute for cats	Get regular veterinary check ups and appropriate exercise.	Labored or difficult breathing; raspy; muffled, congested; rate higher or lower than normal.
Privates	Clean, No discharge, normal size.	If pet can't reach, clean with soft, warm damp cloth	Red, unusual discharge; swollen
Tail	Shiny coat , no lumps, or bumps		Hair loss, open sores, lumps/bumps
Habits	Good energy level and appetitie; doesn't drink water excessively; regular bathroom habits	Feed high quality and age appropriate food; provide fresh, clean water and proper exercise.	Lethargic; loss or increase of appetite / thirst. Change in bathroom habits - more or less frequent "accidents", vomit or diarrhea.

Dental Care – A Clean Mouth Can Mean a Healthy Pet

Brush your cat's teeth regularly for good overall health. Bacteria in the mouth can travel through the bloodstream resulting in damage to the kidneys, heart valves and other organs.

If you notice any of these signs, it's time for a check-up:

- bad breath
- loose teeth
- visible tartar (brownish-yellow stains)
- swelling under the eyes
- difficulty eating
- excessive drooling
- red, irritated, swollen or bleeding gums
- loss of appetite or weight loss
- lethargy or loss of energy

NOTE: Toothaches can make anyone grouchy and result in bad behavior! If your cat suddenly has bad manners, it could be a medical issue.

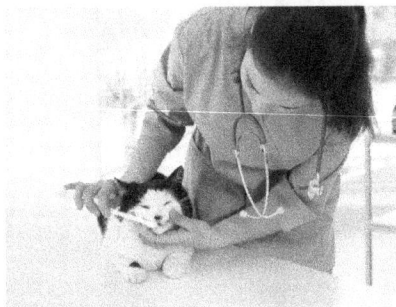

ABCs of Brushing Your Cat's Teeth:

- No one said it would be easy, but you must learn to do this and help your cat get comfortable with you doing so. If kitty is not used to your fingers in her mouth, dip your finger in sodium-free onion-free chicken broth and rub her gums but don't let her nibble your fingers! but don't let him nibble your fingers.
- After a few days of finger massaging, try a pet-specific toothbrush and pet tooth paste. It comes in several flavors so find which one she likes best.
- Coming from behind but over the face place your thumb and index finger at the spot in the check where the upper and lower jaw meet to open mouth. This takes practice and patience. If you brush for 10 seconds on your kitty…you are a rock star! If your pet is reluctant, do just a few teeth, praise her and try again the next day.

Grooming - Keeping up Appearances in Between Trips to the Groomer

Our feline friends need regular grooming because just like you, they feel better when they are clean and healthy. Cats may do much of this themselves since cats are fastidious about their personal hygiene. That being the case, many cats develop fur balls (or bezoars), which are thick, matted tubes of fur that build up in a cat's stomach or intestines. As your cat licks its fur to remove dead hairs from its coat, this loose fur is swallowed, builds up and is then regurgitated or passed through the feces. Sometimes fur balls can cause uncomfortable and dangerous blockages, so by adding fiber to your cat's diet in the form of pumpkin or sweet potato puree (1/2 – 1 teaspoon daily) you can keep fur balls away. Pet stores sell various products and pastes that can help alleviate them as well. The best bet as always is prevention, so fiber and regular grooming by you will lessen the amount of hair swallowed by your cat.

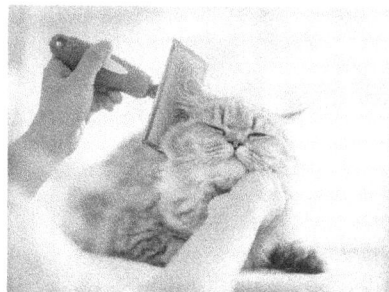

Start when your kitty is young so that grooming becomes a fun thing to do together.

- First brush your cat's coat out thoroughly removing all tangles, mats and snarls. Brush in the same direction that the hair grows with a brush recommended by your groomer or pet store for his particular coat. Brush gently but everywhere -- behind ears, on his belly, tail and legs. Matted fur can cause sores as well as trap heat close to your pet's body.
- There are many types of shampoo, so read labels and don't use ones with products you can't pronounce. Natural is better, and never use a "flea dip" on your kitten, senior cat or a sick cat as they contain harsh chemicals.
- Bathe your cat in a tub of warm water and work shampoo into a good lather avoiding her eyes, nostrils and mouth. Place large cotton balls in her ears to prevent water from getting in, and be sure to rinse off all soap from your cat's skin and fur.
- Remove cotton balls and carefully wipe the insides of both ears with a soft cloth – never a cotton swab which can damage the ear canal.
- Towel dry then brush and thoroughly dry your kitty's coat keeping her warm.
- Trim nails with special cat clippers clippers to prevent them from getting caught in rugs, furniture and humans. ***NEVER have your cat declawed which would be like cutting off your own finger at the first knuckle!***

A NOTE ABOUT DE-CLAWING…Onychectomy is serious surgery! It involves 10 or 20 separate, painful amputations, severing the whole joint including bones, ligaments and tendons and is now illegal in many cities. Complications include chronic pain, nerve damage and recurrent infections. Many Veterinarians struggle with it yet perform the surgery if it is the only way they can save a cat from being euthanized. A cat's claw is so closely adhered to the bone that to remove the claw, the last bone also has to be removed. Think about having the first joint of all your fingers or toes amputated as a comparison – life would not be the same, and it certainly won't be for your kitty. There is no reversal to the surgery. De-clawing is forever!

The feline body is perfectly designed to give it grace and agility. Removing the claws alters the conformation of their feet and deprives a cat of her primary means of defense, leaving her defenseless should she ever escape outdoors. Since she can no longer defend by scratching, your cat may turn to biting and spraying. Some stop using the litter box because the "gravel" hurts tender paws while other cats develop spinal problems since they can no longer walk naturally without their toes. For many it is painful and debilitating.

Scratching posts, cat-nip infused scratching pads, sticky tape on furnishings and nail caps are pain-free alternatives to declawing. Remember, dogs bark and cats scratch – it's what they do, so consider carefully what type of pet best suits your lifestyle BEFORE you make them a part of your home.

Nail Trimming:

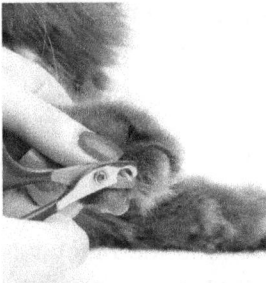

First and foremost, get your cat used to having their paws played with. Touch and gently squeeze paws and look them over from day one.

- Make sure nail clippers are sharp.
- Gently squeeze toe and place an unlit wooden matchstick firmly underneath and clip only the matchstick so that your pet gets used to the sound of the clipper and the pressure applied.
- When ready (this could be an entirely separate day), clip the real thing but pay close attention to the "quick," small blood vessel that runs down the nail and will bleed considerably if cut. On white nails it is dark pink or brown and you want to clip just shy of it. On dark nails take off only a little of the nail at the time until you reach the quick.
- When you look at the cut edge of the nail, you will see a dark center known as the quick when you have cut sufficiently. Being exposed to the air for a couple weeks causes the quick to recede so you can clip again to get the nails shorter without causing bleeding, but…
    - If you cut into the quick, you will hurt your pet and will jeopardize the chance of your pet ever sitting still for a nail trim.
    - you may need to perform first-aid (see page 122) to stop the bleeding; so be prepared to help anytime you do a nail trim.

Anal Glands:

Shaped like a pea, the two anal glands are located just under the skin at the four o'clock and eight o'- clock position under the tail and below the anus. Their nasty smelling fluid is produced by cats to give their stool a unique scent, a way to identify the individual animal. Groomers often express the anal glands during a bath, but if Fluffy has never had a problem, it may not be necessary so consult with your Veterinarian. Learn more on page 114.

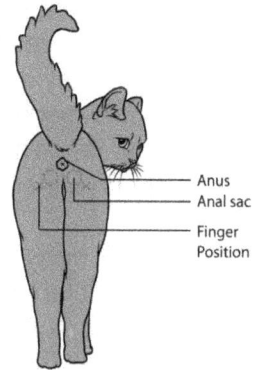

Anus
Anal sac
Finger Position

Parasites: Flea & Tick Free:

Parasites can cause itching, redness and unpleasant skin problems, so keep your cat flea and tick free with preventive treatments recommended by your Veterinarian. Insect-borne diseases can be a serious health risk to people and pets but there is controversy over the safety of applying commercial insecticides, so you may want to consider effective alternatives.

Homeopathic Tip:

- Neem seed oil, from an evergreen tree native to India, has been used as a remedy for a wide variety of skin problems. At 2-3% it is an effective insect repellent although it has a strong scent your pet may not appreciate. Unlike commercial insecticides that can indiscriminately kill insects, neem oil only affects those that chew or suck. When ingested, it disrupts the bug's normal functions making him forget to eat, fly or lay eggs resulting in a diminished population.
- Food grade diatomaceous earth also can keep fleas away from your pets. Diatomaceous earth is a fine powder made from the crushed, fossilized remains of a marine algae. When used in flea prevention, its roughness cuts the flea as it moves causing it to leak water (which the diatomaceous earth absorbs), dehydrating the flea. (You and your pets should be careful and not inhale the diatomaceous earth).

If you discover a tick:

- Slick your cat's hair away from tick and place a cotton ball soaked in rubbing alcohol on the tick. This often causes the tick to back out of your pet for easy removal.
- If that doesn't work, pull tick with tweezers, getting tips close to cat's body without pulling his hair or skin. Do not attempt to suffocate the tick with petroleum jelly or nail polish which results in the tick regurgitating his stomach contents into your kitty. Also, do not try to burn the tick with a match and do not pull a tick with your fingers. By doing so, you'll squeeze its abdomen causing it to regurgitate its stomach contents into your cat!

- Cleanse with peroxide and apply antibiotic ointment. The oxygen in 3% hydrogen Peroxide destroys Lyme disease bacteria so pour it liberally on the skin over bites on light-haired cats (but do keep away from their eyes). For darker-furred cats, it's a good idea to apply the peroxide using an eyedropper. This way you can deliver it directly on the skin and avoid it bleaching out the richer colored fur. It is however much better to have a Lyme Disease-free pet than to worry about a patch of lighter fur. Be aware that if you suspect the tick could be a carrier, save the tick and take it and your cat to the vet for testing. Always be vigilant for signs of infection.

A tick's mouth parts penetrate your cat's skin to suck blood and can leave disease behind, so it's a good idea to keep the tick in a zip lock baggie (after drowning tick in water or alcohol – never crush the tick as that spreads bacteria) in case your cat has a reaction. Your Veterinarian can then determine type of tick and any disease it was carrying.

Know & Vaccinate Against Diseases OR... Get a Titer Test

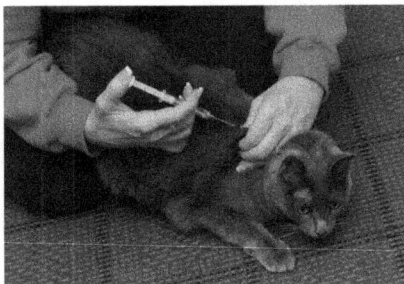

The best protection you can give your dog or cat from certain diseases is to provide regular vaccinations. As puppies and kittens, they receive their immunity from the colostrum in their momma's milk, but once weaned, the antibodies wane so they need injected antigens to create immunity from disease. Think of it as arming your pet's immune system with the correct weapon needed to kill off a specific disease. Research has proven that many vaccinations no longer need to be given annually as protection can last for many years, so discuss with your Veterinarian how infrequently you may safely revaccinate your pet. Humans don't get booster shots annually – actually, many of the vaccinations we receive as children keep us immune for our lifetime, so it's no wonder that dogs and cats, may also not need frequent injections. Too much of a good thing may not be good for your pet when over-vaccination has possible adverse effects (tumors at the sight of the injection, neurological or kidney issues to name a few).

When your cat is due for a booster, discuss titer testing with your Veterinarian. A titer test is a blood sample that when observed on a slide, can determine the level of your cat's immunity to a specific disease. It measures the immune system's preparedness to fight infection and is actually the only proof that your cat has created the antibodies needed to protect itself. Approximately 1 out of every 1,000 pets are non-responders. This means their bodies do not react to the vaccination and fail to create protective antibodies, so getting a vaccination doesn't guarantee that your pet will avoid illness.

In the past titer testing was generally more costly than getting a vaccination, however new technologies are making it more convenient for Veterinarians to test in their offices rather than sending out to a laboratory. Regardless of the cost, if you have a small pet, an older pet or are just concerned about your cat getting too much, a titer test is a good safety precaution, and the extra money you spend on the testing may be saved in the long run if your pet doesn't develop ill effects (tumors, cancer, kidney failure, neurological issues).

For necessary vaccines, consider spacing them out, not having multiple injections at once and NEVER have your cat vaccinated when they are ill or recovering.

What we vaccinate against:
- BACTERIA – Bacteria are single-celled microorganisms that thrive in many different typesof environments. Some varieties live in extremes of cold or heat.
- VIRUS – Viruses are even smaller than bacteria and require living hosts - such as your cats or you --in order to multiply. When a virus enters your cat's body, it invades some of it's cells and takes over their normal function redirecting them to produce the virus.

The Vaccination:
- ANTIGEN – a substance that when introduced into a body triggers production of an antibody by stimulating the cat's immune system. Antigens prime the system to fight.

The Outcome:
- ANTIBODY – protein made by white blood cells that neutralize the effects of toxins; created in response to antigens and make pet immune to a specific disease.

Any medical procedure (including an injection) can have adverse side-effects, so watch your pet for several hours, even days, after any vaccination and get professional medical attention if any of the following arise:

- Fever
- Decrease in social behavior
- Diminished Appetite or Activity
- Sneezing
- Discomfort or swelling at injection site
- Swelling to face or legs
- Vomiting/Diarrhea
- Whole body itching
- Difficulty breathing
- Collapse

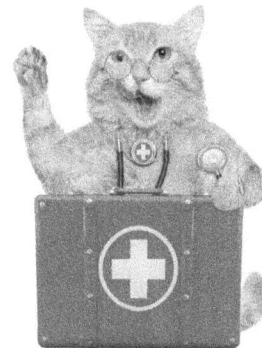

HOMEOPATHIC TIP: Thuja Occidentalis commonly known as Evergreen Conifer Tree, can aid with residual toxicity if given before and after vaccinations. See page 140 under Illness & Injuries to learn more about homeopathic therapies.

Core Vaccinations

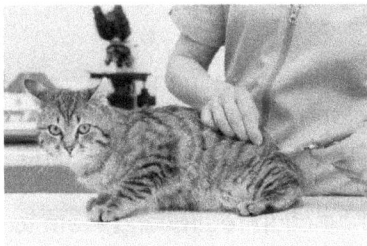

Depending on where you live and what bacteria or viruses are in your region, additional vaccinations may be suggested by your Veterinarian, but as a rule, the following are considered the core inoculations cats should receive with a brief description of the diseases they protect against. Do note, that many illnesses have similar symptoms, so visit your Veterinarian for a professional diagnosis.

Often a combo shot of FVRCP...
- Feline Viral Rhinotracheitis (also known as FHV-1 or Feline Herpes Virus)
- Calicivirus
- Paneleukopenia
- Rabies

CAT DISEASES

Feline Viral Rhinotracheitis and **Calicivirus** are both very contagious upper respiratory infections spread from cat to cat via contact or sneezing.

Symptoms:
- Sneezing & runny nose
- Possibly dirty paws due to wiping their noses
- Occasional mouth sores

Preventive Measures: Vaccinate to prevent.

Panleukopenia is also referred to as Cat Fever or Cat Distemper (canine distemper does not affect cats or vice versa). It is a viral disease spread by direct contact and is similar to the dog strain but cannot cross species. Panleuk can cause a decrease in white blood cells leaving cats susceptible to secondary bacterial infections. It's often fatal in young kittens.

Symptoms:
- Fever Lethargy
- Loss of appetite
- Vomiting and/or diarrhea

Preventive Measures: Vaccinate to prevent.

<u>Feline Urological Syndrome (FUS)</u> is a common problem, yet it's exact cause is unknown. Bad diet, inadequate water intake, bacteria, viruses and stress may play a role as do several common disorders associated with FUS:

- **Cystitis**— inflammation of the lining and wall of the urinary bladder.
- **Infections**— blood or mucus associated with inflamed tissue is a perfect place for bacterial infections.
- **Urethral Blockage**— crystallization of minerals and irritation of the lining of the bladder and urethra can plug up or block the urinary outflow tract. This blockage is life-threatening if not relieved.
- **Uremia**— a life-threatening accumulation of poisonous wastes in the bloodstream. The lack of urination causes a full bladder and this prevents the kidneys from discharging wastes from the body. Unless the blockage is promptly removed, the cat will suffer a painful death. Straining to urinate, depression, weakness, vomiting, and collapse are the signs which, if not corrected, lead to coma and death.

Symptoms:
- Straining to urinate
- Failure to use a litter box (urinating in a sink or bath tub)
- Blood in the urine

What to do: Any of the above symptoms should send you to the Veterinarian. Depending on diagnosis, medication may help or minimize the problem, but some cases require surgical or professionally applied procedures. In order to avoid FUS, be sure to provide plenty of fresh water, feed your cat a balanced diet, keep a clean litter box and provide your pet with exercise.

Tests should be done at your cat's first veterinary visit to find out if she is negative to:

<u>FIV – Feline Immunodeficiency Virus</u> is a widespread viral infection that attacks the immune system rendering your kitty unable to fight infections. It is caused by the same family of viruses that triggers AIDS in humans and has much the same devastating impact on infected cats. It is often referred to as "Kitty AIDS."

It is estimated that less than 15% of the cat population is infected with FIV. The disease is transmitted from cat to cat by blood and saliva. This happens primarily through biting, so outdoor and male cats that fight with other cats are at greatest risk. FIV has also been found in milk and can be transmitted from mother to kitten. Transmission among household cats through normal contact is thought to be unlikely and the disease cannot be transmitted to humans.

The virus does, however, devastate a cat's immune system, stopping it from effectively combating other diseases and infections. Infected cats eventually fall prey to a wide variety of secondary illnesses that overwhelmingly prove fatal. There is no cure, but cats can live for many years – much of it in seeming good health – before succumbing. Cats that do test positive when under 6 months of age should be re-tested after 6 months.

Symptoms: (Please note these can be signs of many diseases so veterinary testing is vital)
- Swollen lymph nodes
- Chronic diarrhea, gingivitis, skin problems
- Anemia/Leukopenia (low red or white blood cell count determined by your Veterinarian)
- Seizures or facial twitching
- Chronic conjunctivitis, glaucoma, cataracts
- Spontaneous abortions or still births

What to do: Veterinary testing and discuss vaccination option. There has been no proven effective treatment for FIV infection. If your cat has no clinical signs, no treatment may be recommended. In this situation, regular follow-up visits to your Veterinarian are important to insure the condition does not progress. If immunodeficiency and secondary infections have developed, your Veterinarian will prescribe antibiotics for bacterial infections, nutritional support, fluid therapy for dehydration and parasite control. Several therapies used to treat people with AIDS have been used in cats with FIV infection with the goal of boosting their immune systems and slowing the progress of the disease. These include the drugs AZT, alpha interferon and bone marrow transplants.

FeLV – Feline Leukemia Virus is a virus that wreaks havoc with the immune system and other organs – a form of cancer of the blood cells transmitted through saliva, tears, blood, urine and feces. Research indicates that feline leukemia is highly contagious among cats of all ages. Current research indicates that it does not affect humans or other species, but a momma cat can pass the FeLV along to her kittens before they are born. Some with strong immune systems can overcome.

Symptoms:
- Loss of appetite
- Vomiting and/or diarrhea
- Respiratory distress
- Neurological abnormalities; progressive weakness
- Anemia (pale gums)
- Jaundice (yellow in the white of the eyes and the gums) Breathing difficulty
- Weight loss
- Recurring chronic illnesses

Preventive Measures: Avoid exposure to infected cats and update vaccinations.

Zoonotic Diseases

Zoonotic diseases can be passed between species, meaning...YOU can get these from being around your pets.

<u>Rabies</u> – Vaccinate or confirm titers to prevent! Rabies is an acute and deadly viral infection of the central nervous system. Although rare in the United States for humans to actually contract rabies, 18,000 Americans each year get shots due to coming in contact with animals that may carry the disease. It is still quite prevalent in Third World Countries.

<u>Toxoplasmosis</u> is an infectious disease found in some farm animals and household pets. Cats are carriers of the disease and can transmit it to people through feces - especially when fecal material is handled or allowed to sit until old and dry. The disease is then either ingested from the fecal matter or it can become airborne and inhaled. Although cats can transmit the disease, they are not the major sources of infection to humans. People are more likely to pick up toxoplasmosis by handling or eating raw meat. Cats contract toxoplasmosis from eating mice and birds, so an outdoor cat stands a greater chance of being exposed or infected.

Symptoms in cats (although often no symptoms are present):
- Lethargy
- Loss of appetite
- Fever

Symptoms in people:
- Mild, flu-like symptoms, but the problem is more serious for pregnant women or immunocompromised individuals. An unborn child of a woman infected during pregnancy may develop birth defects.
- Immunocompromised individuals developing toxoplasmosis usually have a reactivation of a previous infection.

What to do: Do not give away your cat if you are pregnant. Cats should not lose their homes because humans are coming into the world. Rather...be smart. You can prevent the spread of toxoplasmosis by following these simple steps:

- Someone other than a pregnant woman or immunocompromised person should clean the litter box daily as the feces of an infected cat becomes infectious within 36-48 hours.

- Feed cats dry, canned, or thoroughly cooked food and keep them from hunting.

- Cook meat thoroughly to over 151 degrees Fahrenheit. Wash your hands and any thing else that comes in contact with the raw meat such as cutting boards, knives, and the sink.

- Wear gloves when working in the garden or with soil where cats may have left feces, and wash your hands thoroughly afterwards.

- Go to your OB/GYN or medical doctor and have a titer test done to see if you are immune to toxoplasmosis. Then, you can still practice good hygiene, but breathe a sigh of relief and keep your cat in your home and heart.

Giardia - Giardia are one-celled organisms (protozoa) that live in the small intestine of many animals. They attach to the small intestine where they produce disease by taking away nutrients from your pet. The disease, Giardiasis (aka "Beaver Fever" since beavers are known carriers), is found throughout the United States and most places where stagnant water exists. A cat can become infected by eating the cyst form of the parasite when she drinks from a pond, puddle or even a backyard bucket that contains contaminated water. Once the cyst enters your cat's gastrointestinal tract, it releases a trophozoite which whips its hairlike structures (flagella) back and forth for propulsion until it finds a place in your cat's intestine to attach itself to. It then reproduces by dividing, ultimately passing in your cat's feces where it can contaminate the environment and water and infect other animals and people and the cycle continues.

Preventive Measures: Because Giardia is not species-specific, people can get it from their pets or directly from contaminated water sources! Therefore, sanitation is of the utmost importance when caring for your cats. Wear gloves when cleaning up feces, especially diarrhea or vomit from an infected animal, and wash your hands frequently when around your pets. The only sure way to prevent Giardia is to eliminate the source of the infection which is contaminated water as it can survive chlorination as well as frost. Any place water collects should be alleviated if possible such as places where there are puddles or poor drainage. Concrete surface should be cleaned, dried and sealed. Lysol®, ammonia or bleach (1% bleach, 99% water) can be effective decontamination agents, yet due to a protective outer shell, some Giardia survive chlorine treatments.

Signs & Symptoms:
- Diarrhea and/or vomiting
- Weight loss (Since Giardia prevent proper absorption of nutrients and interfere with digestion, your pet may lose weight in spite of eating a hearty meal.)

What to Do: Veterinary care is a must and humans should also get medical attention to get through the discomfort. Most common treatment is the drug Metronidazole (aka Flagyl) which cannot be given to pregnant pets or humans. Usually immunity to Giardia is not acquired after treatment, so contraction of the disease can re-occur. Prevention is always the best medicine, so at home, hiking or on vacation, be sure there is plenty of fresh water for Fluffy and you!

Cat Scratch Fever

Cat scratch fever is a bacterial infection (Bartonella heselae) caused by licks, bites or scratches from a cat or kitten. Symptoms may not appear for several days and may last for several weeks. According to the Center for Disease Control, more than 20,000 cases are reported annually although many more mild cases occur.

Symptoms in humans:
- Pain & swelling at location of bite and lymph nodes
- Malaise
- Fever
- Loss of Appetite

What to Do: Receive medical attention for penicillin or antibiotic therapy.

Ringworm

Ringworm is a fungus, not a worm! It gets its name from the appearance of a ring-shaped rash on the skin that is dry and scaly or wet and crusty with missing patches of hair or fur. Humans can acquire it from dogs and cats, puppies and kittens. Goats, cows, pigs and horses can transfer it to people as well. It can also be obtained from showers, pool surfaces and contaminated clothing. A Wood's Lamp (blue light) will make the fungus glow and determine diagnosis along with a skin biopsy or culture.

Preventive Measures: Prevent contact with infected animals so be on the look-out for signs and symptoms.

Signs & Symptoms:
- Red itchy & raised, scaly patches that may blister and ooze
- On humans, the patches are often redder on the outside with normal skin tone in the center making it appear like a clearly-defined ring.
- On pets, a circular patch of missing fur with a crusty center

What to do: Get pets to their Veterinarian for anti-fungal treatment and humans to their medical professionals! Ringworm is highly contagious!

To care for ringworm:
- Keep skin clean and dry.
- Apply antifungal or drying powders, lotions, or creams that contain miconazole, clotrimazole, or whatever is prescribed by your medical professional.
- Don't wear clothing that rubs against and irritates the area.
- Wash sheets and night clothes, dog and cat bedding every day while infected exists in your household.

Others to be aware of:

Lyme Disease (measles-like eruptions accompanied by muscle aches, nausea and swollen lymph nodes) and **Rocky Mountain Spotted Fever** ('target'-shaped rash bringing with it headache and nausea) are both tick-borne diseases. Keep pets free of parasites and check yourself after hikes. Although humans don't get this one, watch cats for **Cytauxzoonosis**! It comes from the Lone Star and American Dog Tick. Also known as Bobcat Fever, it causes felines to go down fast and they can die within days of being bitten as the infection prevents blood from flowing to tissues resulting in multiple organ failure. Please be reminded that even indoor cats CAN get parasites!

The Importance of Spaying & Neutering

For every human being born 45 kittens are born. How can we possibly provide them all safe and loving forever homes? Due to the frequent heat cycles in cats (every 3 weeks during Kitten Season, March – September), one non-spayed female cat and her offspring can produce 420,000 cats in seven years!

Many animals die giving birth when bred before 6 months of age as they are still babies themselves.

Pet overpopulation is the number one killer of pets! Every 11 seconds a dog or cat is euthanized in the United States. With 80,000 pets born each day versus only 10,000-15,000 people, there will never be enough humans to care for them. Limiting their population growth is the best way to prevent animal homelessness, curb certain diseases, and keep our pets safe.

Spaying and neutering can decrease AGGRESSIVENESS in many pets as hormones no longer rage since the source of their production has been removed. However, your pet still remains protective of his home and family as if he was prior to surgery.

Spay/neuter can decrease SPRAYING (urine marking) particularly by male cats who no longer feel the need to mark their territory. It can also decrease an animal's desire to roam in search of a mate and therefore, your pet stays safely at home. Studies show that 80% of all dogs and cats hit by cars are unneutered males!

Spaying females can lower their risks of mammary and uterine cancer as well as pyometra (an infection of the uterus that can erupt into an emergency situation).

Neutering males can lower prostate issues, so just check with your Veterinarian to find out what age is best to have your pet altered. Most animals go home the same day as surgery and suffer no ill effects (as long as you prevent them from picking at their stitches).

- In brief, SPAYING (ovariohysterectomy) includes the removal of the ovaries, fallopian tubes and uterus. General anesthesia is necessary.

- NEUTERING removes the testicles but will allow your dog to retain his own unique personality. General anesthesia is required, but neuter patients recover more quickly than their female counterparts as neutering is not considered major surgery since it is not performed deep in the abdominal cavity. Non-surgical neutering is in development, so stay tuned to breakthroughs.

Confirm local laws as spay/neuter may decrease the COST OF LICENSING in your area or may actually be mandatory at a certain age for all pets. Low cost clinics and vouchers from humane organizations are available to help those having difficulty paying for spay/neuter surgery. In the long run, the medical cost is much cheaper than caring for a litter of puppies or kittens.

Common Myths Dispelled

Spaying/Neutering DOES NOT make your cat fat or lazy – lack of exercise and overfeeding does.

Cats DO NOT need to have one litter to settle down. Having a litter will not improve your cat's health or change her personality. Actually, pregnancy and nursing can sometimes cause pets to become tired & irritable.

DON'T leave your pet unaltered so that your child can see the "miracle of birth." Most animals hide when giving birth and even if you find good homes for your litter, you may deny homes to those that have already been born. There are plenty of videos available to learn these life lessons.

CARING FOR A NEONATE: Your Newborn Kitten

Red Flags
Seek IMMEDIATE medical attention if your kitten is:
- Coughing
- Sneezing
- Gagging
- Wheezing

Has:

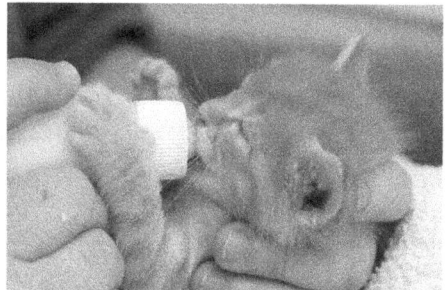

- Diarrhea
- Vomiting
- Loss or increased appetite
- Change in behavior

Is:

- Twitching abnormally
- Straining to urinate or defecate
- Tiring easily
- Breathing heavily
- Bleeding from any part of the body

Milestones:

Week #1   Weight should double

Week #2   Eyes open! If they seem weepy or pus-filled, gently wipe with a warm, wet, soft cloth but do not pry open. Let eyes open naturally. Fur babies can hear!

Week #3   Crawling on all fours! Kittens ears start to stand up at this point.

Week #4   Kittens begin playing with each other and start to develop teeth. Ouch! The transition begins to wet food.

Week #6   Dry food is on the menu and eye color may begin changing from blue (although true color doesn't settle in until about the 3rd month).

Week #8   Kittens should weigh 2 lbs. and are big enough to be spayed or neutered. They will look like mini-versions of full grown cats and will have all their baby teeth. Check with your veterinarian as to when best spay or neuter your feline friend.

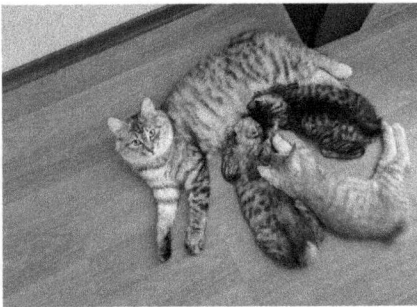

Warmth

Keeping your newborn kitten warm is of supreme importance. Neonates haven't yet developed the ability to keep themselves temperate so they are very dependent on you for their climate control. Being too hot or too cold can be a true medical emergency!

Cleanliness

No animal can stay healthy if he is not kept clean. Kittens will soil themselves. If you have a litter, the animals will groom each other, and if feces, old food or mucous is stuck in their fur, the other animal will ingest it and become ill.

Bathe kittens carefully in warm water using kitten shampoo taking care not to get water or shampoo in their eyes, ears, nose or mouth. Always use species specific products (do not use soaps, flea preventatives, or anything for cats that is made for dogs). After the bath, wrap the cat in a towel and dry thoroughly. This also creates a loving bond between you and the animal.

Feeding

Never feed a newborn when he or she is cold as they are prone to aspiration pneumonia, gut motility problems and won't be able to properly digest their food. Warm fluids should be administered until the animal is warm enough to be fed.

An eye dropper or bottle with nipple will be needed for a kitten who does not have a mom to nurse her. Use a sewing needle or a 16-18 gauge hypodermic needle to first pierce the tip of the nipple. Too large of an opening in the nipple could cause the kitten to aspirate the fluid into the lungs. Too small of an opening will prevent her from getting the nutrition she needs.

Before you begin feeding, thoroughly clean the bottle and nipple in hot water and wash your hands with antibacterial soap. Gently open the kitten's mouth with the tip of your finger and gently slip the nipple in. You will feel a vacuum effect when she gets the nipple into suckle mode and will probably then hold on enthusiastically. Keep the bottle at a 45 degree angle with light tension on the bottle to prevent air from getting into the young one's stomach.

If the kitten refuses the bottle, try rubbing her forehead or back to simulate how her mom would clean her and encourage her to nurse.

Let her suck at her own pace but do not overfeed – animals generally let you know when they've had enough. Each feeding can take 20-30 minutes via the bottle. If the kitten is choking, immediately and carefully hold her upside down. Below is a good rule of thumb to follow for kittens:

Newborn to 1 week old	1 – 2 Tablespoons
1 – 2 weeks	3 Tablespoons
2 – 3 weeks	4 – 5 Tablespoons
3 – 4 weeks	6 Tablespoons

Make only enough formula that will be used within 48 hours. For canned formula, freeze any leftovers in an ice cube tray and thaw only what you need for each additional feeding. Pet Ag makes KMR® (Kitten Meal Replacement) for kittens. Cow's milk is not a good substitute for young cats.

Kittens sometimes need to be encouraged to defecate. Momma cats help their kids along by licking their babies' urogenital openings to stimulate urination and defecation. If you are playing the role of mom, use a cotton ball dampened with warm water to wipe the areas. Remember to wash your hands before and after handling neonates. Always use clean towels and don't believe the old wives tale about newspaper being sterile, unless it is non-inked! The ink from newspaper can be toxic and easily absorbed through the animal's skin.

Like humans, felines are about 70% water and need to stay well-hydrated.
Daily test their hydration by gently pulling up on the skin at the nape of their neck and releasing. This is called the skin tugor test, and a well-hydrated animal's skin will snap back quickly – within one second or less. If the skin stays in a peak or takes 2-3 seconds to return to position, give fluids through a needle-less syringe or eye dropper and seek medical attention immediately.

At Four Weeks
Kittens should be introduced to the litter box! Place kittens in their box after each meal.

If nothing happens, gently rub the lower abdomen and use a warm wet cotton ball on their genitals and rectum, just enough to stimulate activity. Don't cause irritation to their tender skin. Kittens should be defecating at least once a day. If tummy is stretched tight or kitten appears to strain with no results, you have a constipated kitten (see section on Constipation page 147).

Also at four weeks, kittens should now be fed every 4-6 hours transitioning to wet/canned/soft food. They should also start drinking water on their own at this time. Often kittens start biting at their bottle nipple when they are ready for this change. To encourage your kitten or puppy to eat wet food or mix KMR® with the soft food into a porridge-like consistency and serve off a spoon or your finger until they are ready to plunge into their food bowl. At this stage of the game they still lack coordination and often fall head first into their food bowls so be prepared to clean your little one after each meal and don't be surprised if he or she treats you to spells of diarrhea during this weaning period.

At Six Weeks
Another food transition and yes…more diarrhea comes at 6 weeks of age when you should wean your kitten from the soft food to dry food. For the first week, mix canned and dry together and gradually reduce the amount of wet. Make sure you are using kitten kibble so that the bits are small enough to be chewed by teeny weenie teeth. By 8 weeks the kibble size may be increased, as long as they are able to chew the bits comfortably – you do not want a choking incident.

Socializing
Emotional and physical closeness is important to kittens. Let them snuggle, pet them as much as you can, and try out various toys to find out which ones stimulate their brain power and develop their motor skills. As they reach 6-8 weeks old, they should be out of their crates more safely exploring the world WITH YOU. Let them walk about a bedroom or other smaller room where you can keep a watchful eye. Make sure cords and strings are out of paws and claws reach but let them use their muscles and gain control of their motor skills while smelling the scents of home. Make sure there are no chemicals or cleaning products on the floor, and watch that they don't slip between furniture or escape from the house completely.

There is nothing as cute as a bundle of fur licking your face with that distinct kitten breath and a soft round tummy. It can turn any grown-up into a cooing human child. Rediscovering the world through an inquisitive kitten's eyes is a delight, but it's also important to note how first experiences must be good and positive for your young one. A hand or voice raised in anger or a lack of experiences with others can allow an adorable kitten to grow into a hissy cat of questionable. From the moment your kitten enters your life, you must socialize her to become a friendly and confident cat.

People and the Human Touch

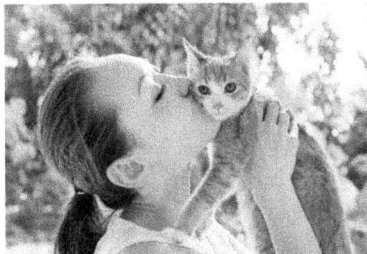

People are number one on the list as far as "what" you should desensitize your pet to according to Vernon, New York Veterinarian Deb Eldredge, "and people of different sizes, ages, sexes, people with hats, people with facial hair." She insists that every new thing should be positive.

Pet parent Norma Chavez says, "I took a Pet First-Aid Class and learned the importance of doing a weekly head-to-tail check-up on my pet. Bella became so used to me touching her that it's now easy if she gets hurt, needs a bath or has to be touched for any reason. She'll let me feel around and even put an ice pack on her. I never had a pet before that was used to this."

Sights, Sounds and Smells

At home, pull out the vacuum cleaner, ring the doorbell, clap your hands and play the stereo. Pop some corn or percolate coffee with your furry angel by your side.Get her used to her crate and carrier. Place soft blankets, toys and treats in it in the house so that it becomes a safe refuge. Then slowly take your kitty in her carrier for short car rides and to the vet, even when she doesn't have an appointment. Sit in the waiting room with kitty next to you in her carrier, feeding her treats. After a few moments, leave and go home. This allows her to take in the sights and smells and keeps going to the veterinarian a good experience.

The Carrier/Crate

The purpose of a cat carrier/crate is really three-fold…it is a den to keep the animal safe, helps with potty training and allows cats to develop a tolerance for car rides and going to the Veterinarian!

Since young cats aren't yet equipped to control their body temperature, placing a heating pad on a low setting in the carrier conserves the warmth keeping the animal comfortable. The heating pad should be well wrapped in a towel with another towel on top of it – the puppy or kitten should NEVER make contact with the pad directly and should be used only until the animal is about 4 weeks old. Constantly recheck your heating pad for safety sake!

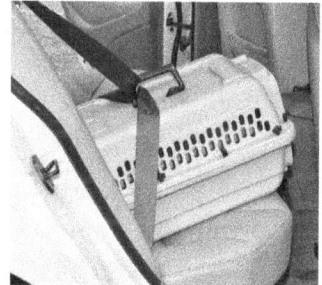

Carriers/crates should be kept in draft-free locations and the bedding will need to be changed several times daily. By four weeks when they are transitioning to wet food, start putting the kitten in her litter box with you immediately after each meal to train them where to go.

CAT SAFETY

You can't keep your cat in a plastic bubble – life happens, and statistics show that 9 out of 10 pets are going to experience an emergency at some point during their lifetime, so don't be caught not knowing what to do. Although tips are provided in this section, more detailed first-aid techniques are available in the back of this book to walk you through what to do when the worst happens.

Beforehand, make your cat's environment as safe as possible and always keep your eyes wide open. When you have a pet, you have a furry toddler for life, and…one who possesses a kitty sense of smell! This means that even when you may feel items are put away, they are never truly out of "paws and claws reach" if they smell good enough to get. Our pets can smell a whole lot better than we can – statistics show their sense of smell is from 1,000 to 1,000,000 times better than ours! This means that an item of no concern to us has a virtual rainbow of scents to our pet, and if tempting enough, your cat might seek it out.

Down on all fours
Look at life from your pet's perspective. What may be perfectly tidy at 5'4", 6'2" or wherever you stand…is a whole different world at 6" - 10" off the floor. Anything on the floor is fair game, so besides teaching cats "no" and "leave it," it is up to you to limit the dangers they can encounter.

Feline Foibles
The following are some of the many common items to keep out of paws and claws reach in basic home scenarios:

Living Room
- Electric cords
- TV – remote controls can look like toys
- Stereos – can be deafeningly loud to animals' sensitive hearing
- Falling knick knacks, pictures, lamps
- Sharp coffee table edges
- Cords from blinds and draperies – choking and entanglement issues
- Rug chewing – result in intestinal blockages
- Rocking chairs – can catch tails and paws
- Fireplace including smokeless logs from which the sawdust can cause a bowel obstruction and lighter fluid poisoning
- Heating units/vents
- Window Screens – are they secure in ALL rooms of the house, so that your kitty sunning herself on a sill won't fall out?

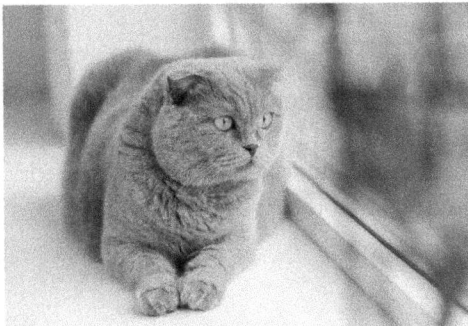

Kitchen

According to the Pet Poison Helpline® (800) 213-6680,
the Top 10 Kitchen Toxins are:

1) Chocolate
2) Grapes, raisins, currants
3) Xylitol found in sugar-free gum & candy
4) Fatty table scraps
5) Onions & garlic
6) Compost
7) Human Medications
   - NSAIDs (Advil, Aleve & Motrin for example)
   - Acetaminophen (Tylenol)
   - Antidepressants (Effexor, Cymbalta, Prozac, Lexapro)
   - ADD/ADHD Medications (Adderall, Ritalin, Concerta)
   - Benzodiazepines & Sleep Aids (Xanax, Klonopin, Ambien, Lunesta)
   - Birth Control (Estrogen, Estradiol, Progesterone)
   - ACE Inhibitors (Zestril, Altace)
   - Beta Blockers (Tenormin, Toprol, Coreg)
   - Thyroid Hormones (Armour desiccated thyroid, Synthroid)
   - Cholesterol Lowering Agents (Lipitor, Zocor, Crestor)
8) Macadamia Nuts
9) Cleaning Supplies
10) Unbaked bread dough & alcohol, both of which can lead to alcohol poisoning

But also watch out for...

- Stove/Oven – hot burners, long after they've been turned off!
- Electric cords & outlets – can be enticing if splashed by food items
- Cleaners
- Other pantry items – many are fatal to pets (see page 213 for list of common poisonous foods) Oxygen absorbers placed in meat packing containers
- Knives and sharp tools
- Cabinet doors/refrigerator/dishwasher – make sure pets don't get closed in tight quarters and food gets dropped – pets can be stepped on

Bathroom

- Medications -- #1 cause of poisoning in our pets! Prescription & over the counter.
- Medical Marijuana (but of course this could be "stashed" elsewhere in the home)
- Cleaners
- Falling in or drinking out of toilet containing chemicals
- Electric outlets and appliances
- Candles
- Standing water in tubs or showers which could be a drowning hazard
- Dental Floss

Bedroom

- Drapery and blind cords
- Anything that can fall – knick knacks, pictures, mirrors, television sets, items from shelves
- Bed collapse – if pet sleeps underneath
- Rug or blanket chewing
- Any medications in nightstand
- Batteries (such as from hearing aids or other appliances)
- Getting closed in cabinets/closets
- Children's toys which could be anywhere in the house
- Shoe laces, hair ribbons and other such pieces of clothing

Garage & Outdoor Areas

- Paints, paint removers, cleaners of all types
- Insecticides & fertilizers
- Car engines – always tap on in cold months as an animal could be keeping warm near the engine and check before you back out!
- Barbeques – charcoal, lighter fluid, matches and the flame itself
- Pools/Spas/Fountains – drowning is always a concern; fenced off or ALWAYS supervise pets! What about chlorine and other chemicals? If pet gets into or drinks water containing chemicals, either could be very bad news.
- Sprinkler systems and outdoor electrical wiring
- Hot concrete and other surfaces
- Trash – secured lids
- Wildlife – pet friendly deterrents may be needed to keep them away; motion sensor lighting & sprinklers; picking up trash & dropped fruit to avoid raccoons or opossums; citronella and pet-safe preventives from mosquitoes, fleas and ticks

While this is not a complete list, it is a great starting point for you. Please take time to review your entire home for potential issues and problems.

Besides locations, each season has its own inherent dangers to our pets. Fun-in-the-sun, splash-in-the-pool, throw-one-on-the-barbie time can be dangerous for your pets unless you keep a watchful eye. Cookouts can result in burned paws while summer-time foods like burgers, franks and fried chicken can cause feline pancreatitis (an inflammation of the organ that is the body's source of insulin and enzymes necessary for digestion).

Spring & Summer

Warmer weather, blooming plants and buzzing insects can spell trouble for your pets but also note that depending where you live, winter hazards may still apply.

Observe your cats whenever outdoors. Dangers exist everywhere, but good pet parenting can prevent disasters and fix up minor injuries.

Insects

If your playful pussy cat gets stung by a bee, scrape away the stinger if you actually see it in her fur coat (or on her nose, lip or paw). Pulling the stinger with fingers or tweezers could rupture the poison sac allowing the toxin to enter your cat's body. Next administer 1 mg Benadryl® (Diphenhydramine) per pound of your pet's body weight, and apply a cold pack for short periods at a time (a bag of frozen peas works well) to any swelling. Remove ice pack frequently so as not to cause frostbite to the tissue or discomfort to your cat in general. If the swelling is severe or if any breathing difficulties develop, get to your Veterinarian at once! (Reference page 128 for more information)

Rising Temperatures

Be sure pets have plenty of shade and water as it warms up but realize colder days sometimes revisit. Know weather patterns and stay alert to your regional changes.

Although much more tolerant of heat than dogs, cats don't sweat! Panting works like an evaporative cooling system bringing in cool air only if there is any. An air-conditioned house is safest for your pet, but the next best thing is a well shaded porch with a fan or misting system. Provide fresh water all day long making sure that outside bowls remain in the shade even when the sun moves in the late afternoon.

Tap water and many bottled waters are full of contaminants that a simple filter can remove. Heavy metals, chlorine and pharmaceuticals are just some of the toxins found in water. They can affect your pet's skin, coat and overall health! Always, always use either a stainless steel, glass or ceramic bowl for water. Plastic bowls can leach toxins into the water so avoid them altogether. Place outside food bowls in a pan containing a few inches of water to keep ants at bay. Notice the sun's patterns in regards to shade as well. Trees may not have grown their full complement of leaves by the time the sun is burning down.

Hot concrete and asphalt can burn precious paws!

When out for a car ride, if your cat cannot go with you on every stop, leave her at home in a comfortable environment. Even with windows open, a parked car can quickly reach more than 150°F resulting in heat stroke, permanent brain damage or death to your pet. Never EVER leave your cat unattended in the car for even a few minutes. Additionally, they could be cat-napped or badly injured by shattered glass if someone tries to break into your car.

Plants

It is important to learn which plants in your yard are poisonous. Besides the toxins that flowers, bulbs, leaves and stems contain, thorns can cause pain and infections. Many fruits and vegetables can also be problematic. Remember, canine, feline and human bodies are not the same, and just because we eat it does not make it safe for our pets. Although less problematic in cats than in dogs, still keep grapes and raisins, onions and chives, seeds and fruit pits away from Fluffy – the stone pit or seed in fruits such as peaches and plums contain an arsenic or cyanide-like substance that can prove fatal.

According to the Pet Poison Helpline®, the 10 most dangerous plants to our pets are:
- Autumn Crocus – all parts
- Azalea – all parts
- Cyclamen – all parts
- Daffodils – especially bulbs
- Diffenbachia – leaves and stems
- Kalanchoe – all parts including vase water are toxic
- Lilies – true lilies…Tiger, Asiatic, Easter and Japanese Snow can be fatal to cats! Others may cause milder symptoms.
- Oleander – all parts, even the water in a vase, are toxic
- Sago Palm – all parts but seeds most deadly
- Tulips/Hyacinths – especially bulbs

Find a more comprehensive list on page 212.

Also take caution with what you put on your plants…fertilizers, insecticides and even yard trimmings can be fatal if ingested by your pet. Have phone numbers accessible for your Veterinarian and Poison Control (ASPCA Animal Poison Control # - 888-426-4435), and the Pet Poison Helpline (855) 886-7965. Know where your nearest animal emergency center is located. In an emergency, you don't want to be looking up directions!

Try this pet friendly weed killer you can make yourself:
> 1 Gallon White Vinegar
> 2 Cups Epsom Salts
> ¼ Cup Dawn® Dish Soap (the original blue works best)
> Mix and spray in the morning after the dew has evaporated.
> By dinner time…weeds are gone!

Also realize organic fertilizers can be deadly if consumed. Blood meal is flash frozen blood that has been dried and ground but is still found tasty to pets. Often it is infused with iron resulting in a toxic overdose if kitty licks some off her paws, while bone meal is made from animal bones that have been ground to powder. That meaty taste is inviting but when ingested, can form a large concrete-like ball in your pet's stomach which requires surgical removal.

Water Fun

Don't assume your pet can swim! Many animals drown each year, so install a fence or pool alarm and teach your furry friends how to get out of the pool by guiding them to the steps or a ramp. Review this lesson often, and if you take your cat to the lake or on a boat, put her in a life vest and watch paws for fish hooks, sharp rocks and other dangers. Safely store all chemicals associated with your pool and outdoor activities such as chlorine, pH, diatomaceous earth for filters and do not let the pool become your pet's drinking bowl since you add these chemicals to the water. Remember that pool toys can make a pet curious causing him to jump in unattended or even get entangled or choke on chewed pieces. It pays to know cat first-aid every season of the year, because harm can and could happen to your pet. Be prepared for your cat's!

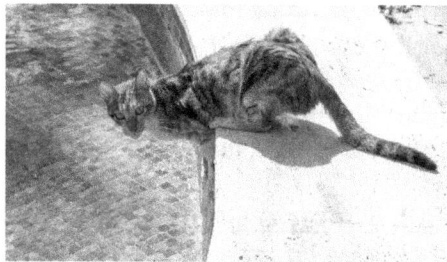

By being an always alert pet parent, you can keep the fun flowing while keeping your furry kids out of harm's way, so open your eyes to impending hazards that could put on the brakes to summer-time fun.

Parasites, Insects & Snakes

Control fleas and ticks and keep your cats well groomed, but don't shave long-haired cats down to the skin as their fur insulates from the heat and prevents sunburn. Learn cat first-aid for bee stings and insect bites. Hot weather brings out rattlesnakes. Your best safety device is keeping control of your cat by keeping her indoors or in a screened patio. Limit the rodent population in your yard by removing ivy and piles of wood since where there are mice, there are snakes to eat them! Should your pet get bitten by a rattlesnake, keep him calm and immediately transport him to an animal care center. See pages 128 - 136 before you need to know what you must do for snake bites and bee stings.

Paws Off

Keep insect repellents and sunscreens out of reach. If ingested by your pet, these products can result in neurological problems, vomiting and diarrhea. This includes citronella candles and other such items.

Make sure your pets keep paws and claws off matches and lighter fluid. Although cats are less likely to consume items than dogs, you never know if you are lucky enough to have a more-than-average curious cat on your hands. Some matches contain chlorates which if ingested can damage her red blood cells, cause difficulty breathing or even kidney problems. Lighter fluid can irritate the skin, cause gastrointestinal, central nervous system, and pulmonary distress.

Also, since the hot days have arrived, make sure your pet doesn't walk on any surfaces that could burn his paws. If it's too hot for your bare feet, it's too hot for kitty's four paws! It's rare, but cats can actually leave behind prints when they sweat out the paws. Be aware of the dangers of heat stroke and make sure your pets have plenty of cool, fresh water and shade to retreat to. Getting over heated can result in permanent brain damage and death to your cat, so never, never, never leave her alone in a parked car -- even for a short time. It only takes a few minutes (with the windows rolled down which can present a danger in itself) for the car to heat to deadly temperatures. See Heatstroke on page 165.

When the day is done, you'll be happy to have taken extra care so that your cat will be around to spend many long and happy years by your side.

Fall, Winter & Colder Days to Come
A sudden change of schedule can lead to stress in your cat and can cause behavioral problems. Extra attention and a new friend may be the solution.

After a summer of getting lots of attention from their favorite boy or girl, your cat may not be herself when the kids dash off on the first day of the new school year. The sudden disruption to her schedule and quality time may cause your cat to eat too much, not want to eat at all or start eating strange objects such as plants, dirt, toys or clothing. This can result in vomiting, diarrhea and skin problems to name a few. Now is the time to give your four-legged family member some extra attention and to sharpen up on your pet first-aid and CPR skills because no matter how hard you try...life happens.

As leaves begin to fall, gardening tools and other sharp objects may get hidden. Look around to be sure that nothing can cut precious paws if you have a cat who roams the green earth with you..

Don't leave pets outdoors when the temperature drops. All cats are safer indoors, except when taken out for exercise. Regardless of the season, shorthaired, very young, or old pets should never be left outside without supervision. Short-coated Cats may feel more comfortable wearing a sweater, even indoors, as temperatures drop.

Warm engines in parked cars attract cats and small wildlife who may crawl up under the hood to get warm. To avoid injuring any hidden animals, bang on your car's hood to scare them away before starting your engine.

Salt and other chemicals used to melt snow and ice can irritate the pads of your cat's feet if she goes out for a stroll. Wipe paws gently with a damp towel before your cat licks them and irritates his mouth. Antifreeze is a deadly poison, but it has a sweet taste that attracts animals. Take care to quickly wipe up spills and store antifreeze (and all household chemicals) out of reach. Better yet, use antifreeze-coolant made with propylene glycol; if swallowed in small amounts, it will not hurt pets.

New Year's Resolutions for Your Cat

I RESOLVE TO:
Do a weekly head-to-tail check-up of my cat and really get acquainted with his habits so that I can discover a small problem before it becomes a nightmare.

Schedule a visit with our Veterinarian to discuss any findings and have our vet do his or her own examination, run tests, give any necessary vaccinations and let me know of any special needs my cat may have.

Check into veterinary insurance or have a "Plan B" (credit card or separate bank account) so that if my cat needs medical care, I will be able to provide it.

Sign-up for a CAT FIRST-AID & CPCR Class and have a CAT FIRST-AID KIT (see page 99) on hand, so that I can help my best friend before veterinary care is available.

Cut out table scraps (except for carrots, bananas, string beans and other cat-friendly human foods) and keep my cat well exercised. Sometimes the best exercise for a cat is adopting another cat, and that way we save a life too!

Brush my cat's teeth (or wipe the teeth and gums) at least every other day to prevent bacteria from travelling through my pet's bloodstream. See page 42.

Make sure my cat has a microchip and identification on him at all times and keep her safely indoors.

Provide my cat with a comfortable place to sleep in a warm, draft-free area.

Give my cat at least as much unconditional love as she gives me and spend good quality time with her for that is the greatest joy of being a Cat Parent!!!

VALENTINE'S DAY

Life is Like a Box of Chocolates...Unless You Are a Cat!

A study published in the 2006 Journal of Agricultural and Food Chemistry determined that chocolate is the third highest antioxidant source consumed in the U.S. following coffee and tea. According to Mark Stibich, PhD, "Chocolate is made from plants, which means it contains many of the health benefits of dark vegetables. These benefits are from flavonoids, which act as antioxidants which protect the body from aging caused by free radicals, which can cause damage that leads to heart disease. Dark chocolate contains a large number of antioxidants (nearly 8 times the number found in strawberries), and flavonoids help relax blood pressure and keep cholesterol from gathering in blood vessels."

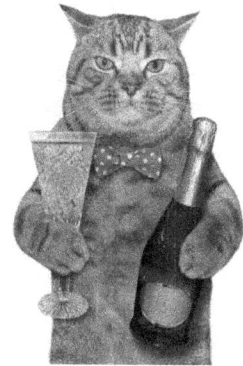

Sounds good so far, but the benefits do not apply to the feline species! According to the ASPCA, its Animal Poison Control Center hotline receives an increased volume of calls from worried pet parents around Halloween, Christmas, Valentine's Day, Easter and Mother's Day, all holidays where candy is abundant. The problem isn't just the fat chocolate contains, but even worse, the caffeine-like substance known as theobromine a naturally occurring stimulant found in the cocoa bean. An animal that has ingested too much chocolate can experience rapid heart rate, vomiting, diarrhea, seizures and death. The only good news is that it takes a fairly large amount of Theobromine to cause a toxic reaction in your pet. However, do realize that every animal is different and some are much more sensitive to toxins than others meaning they can suffer ill effects on even the smallest amount of a substance.

So how much is too much chocolate for your pet? The darker the chocolate, the more dangerous! White chocolate causes the least harm since it contains almost no cocoa and only 1mg of Theobromine per ounce. Milk chocolate, the most common form, contains 60mg per ounce which means: one ounce of milk chocolate per pound of body weight can be toxic! For example: 1/2 pound for an 8 lbs. cat would make her very ill or worse. The chocolate generally found in chocolate chip cookies, semi-sweet chocolate, contains an even higher Theobromine concentration, so less than one ounce per pound your pet weighs can make her just as sick. Theobromine is found in still higher levels in dark chocolate, cocoa powder and bakers chocolate as well as cocoa mulch which often adorns potted plants and flower beds.

Once swallowed, there is no specific antidote for chocolate poisoning, so if you suspect your cat has consumed chocolate, get to the vet at once! Veterinarians do not recommend cat parents inducing vomiting at home. Not always successful on cats even by trained professionals, this is a task best left up to your vet using cat-specific meds So like Forrest Gump always said, "Life is like a box of chocolates. You never know what you're going to get." And for your cat...it will never be a good thing, so NO CHOCOLATE FOR FLUFFY! Also, since you never know what unexpected events will be thrown your way, be prepared by having a well-stocked pet first-aid kit (page 99) along with the knowledge of what to do to help your pet in any kind of emergency.

Fourth of July Fireworks

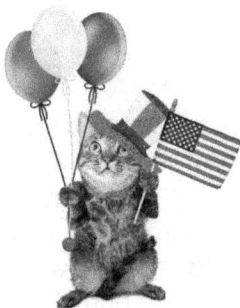

The weeks before and after the Fourth of July are among the busiest at animal shelters across the country. Shelters fill up with strays often making staff have to choose which other animals must be euthanized to make room for the sudden influx. Loud booms and flashing fireworks make humans "oooooo" and "awwww", but they chase our cats from the safety of their homes (not to mention the harm they bring to birds and other wildlife). Escaped animals become disoriented and end up miles away from those who love them, and those are the lucky cats who get picked up and taken to shelters. Many more meet their fate by running frantically into the path of a car.

Be a responsible pet parent making sure to provide a safe environment for your four-legged best friends. Although you may be tempted to bring them along to enjoy the festivities, think again, and follow a few rules so that your cat will be safe and happy when the fifth of July rolls around.

Indoors
Close the drapes and turn on a radio or television to mask any noise and distract the cat's attention from the pops and bangs. Triple check that all doors, windows and gates are secure, and if your pet is easily agitated, make sure someone stays with her during the festivities.

Outdoors
Enjoy your cookout, but keep your cats on their normal diet. Burgers, fries, salty chips, and fried chicken can all upset your cat's stomach while fats from an abundance of these foods can result in pancreatitis. Alcoholic beverages can result in a coma or respiratory failure. Chocolate can be lethal.

If your cat goes outdoors, keep her safe from water hazards.

Keep cats far away from sparklers and firecrackers. One spark on precious fur and you'll need an emergency trip to the Veterinarian. Do not let paw, snout or any part of your furry friend get close as the results could be deadly.

Back-to-School Tips

Things to keep in mind that can help the animals in your household adjust and stay safe:

When the school bell rings, don't let your cat go back to school too. A lonely kitty may want to tag along. Keep your cat confined (especially if she is an outdoor cat) when children leave for school, and if you drive, don't take the pets with you. Animals learn quickly and may find their own way to school later on resulting in them becoming lost or injured. For severe separation anxiety, place the t-shirt your child slept in the night before in your pet's bed -- as long as he doesn't rip it to shreds, it will make her feel like her boy or girl is there with her.

Now that mom or dad may be experiencing a little "empty nesting," it's a great time to spend extra quality time with the family Cat. She'll enjoy extra pets, grooming sessions and a few new toys of her own!

If your cat is seeming bored with the kids away, consider adopting a second cat to keep her company. They will play and exercise together and you will have saved a life.

Pets are part of the family too, so make sure you focus extra attention on them when their world has suddenly been turned upside down by their humans' change of schedule.

Halloween

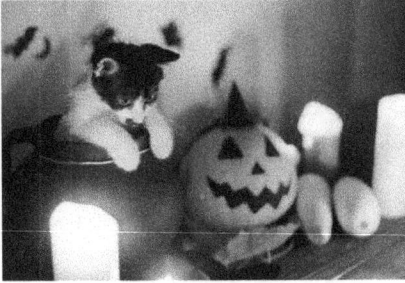

Things that go bump in the night shouldn't include your pets, so follow a few simple tips to make sure Howl-o-ween won't be scary or dangerous for your felines!

PREVENT A HOUDINI ACT by knowing where your cats are at all times. Many felines get scared by the shrieks of ghosts & goblins on the streets or coming to their doors and they dart into the path of cars. Others are scared by masked and caped individuals moving towards them. Keep cats in a quiet back room.

AVOID THE KISS OF DEATH from items ingested. Candy wrappers can cause intestinal blockages and chocolate can be fatal to cats. If you're putting out creepy treats with grapes or raisins masquerading as "eyeballs," make sure your pets do not get them as they can cause kidney failure. Keep plastic toothpicks that adorn festive cupcakes also out of reach, and take care that your pets can't chew or become entangled in wires or electric cords. Ensure cats steer clear of candles haunting the family jack o'lantern as well as fake spider webs and spray string, all of which can burn, choke or cause harm if ingested.

IF YOUR CAT LOOKS MISERABLE...SHE PROBABLY IS! Unless Fluffy is truly comfortable in a costume, her own furry birthday suit might be a better choice. A festive bandana or collar might just fit the bill. Pets aren't used to wearing elastic and definitely don't like masks covering their eyes or nose, so think of your four-legged friend. Is that photo op worth them being uncomfortable? Should you have a cat willing to "dress up," make sure the costume doesn't have beads or strings which they may chew on, and never leave your cat unattended in a costume!

EVIL LURKS IN THE NIGHT, and some people, taking advantage of the anonymity of costumes, partake in malicious pranks targeting black cats, dogs and other animals. Even if you don't normally do so, please, please, please keep your pets in the house on Halloween night. If you see anything suspicious regarding the treatment of an animal, immediately call your local animal control or police department. See if your city has its own animal cruelty task force.

And remember...September and October can still be very HOT in some locations! Make sure your pets have plenty of shade and water. Never leave them unattended in a parked car and be certain that pet carriers and even rooms in your house are cool with good ventilation for your pets.

Thanksgiving

Giving your cats a small nibble of white-meat turkey is okay, just be sure it's boneless and fully cooked. Bones can splinter and dark meat, greasy skin, gristle and gravies can cause severe stomach upsets and pancreatitis in your four-legged friends for which there is no cure! The inflammation to the pancreas (the organ responsible for insulin and enzyme production vital to digestion) must resolve on its own during a period of hospitalization, administration of IV fluids, medication and round-the-clock monitoring for life-threatening complications.

Sweet potato, cooked carrots and green beans are also okay treats if they aren't coated in butter, salt and spices.. Pumpkin puree, although beneficial to a pet suffering from fur balls, constipation or diarrhea, can cause concern if ingested in the form of pumpkin pie or pie mix due to the added sugar, spices and other ingredients. Also, don't overdue pumpkin, as it is a remedy for constipation and too much
can give your pet the runs.

Although sage makes stuffing taste yummy, it contains essential oils and resins that can cause pets to suffer stomach upset and possible depression of the central nervous system, so be sure to keep this herb out of reach.

If you're letting yeast dough rise on the counter, make sure Fluffy doesn't come near. Raw dough in a feline tummy continues to ferment and can result in alcohol poisoning!

Family gatherings bring relatives and friends who may not be as pet savvy as you! Politely give guests a few rules about closing doors and gates behind them so that your precious pets do not escape. Provide a safe place for toothpicks that may be used with hors d'oeuvres, as once dropped on the floor with the aroma of meats and cheeses, these sharp objects become desirable to our pets and can cause puncture and choking injuries.

Be sure to safely tuck away bones, foils and plastic wraps from your pets. The food remnants on these items will make them hard to resist and could cause obstructions, choking incidents and even suffocation to your cat.

The holiday season means lots of cameras, radios and other battery-operated electronics. Please don't leave batteries lying around. If swallowed, they can cause choking or obstruction; if punctured, the chemicals in alkaline batteries can cause burns to the mouth and esophagus.

Finally, holidays often translate to candies and sweets. Read Chocolate Toxicity on page 176, but also realize the wrappers and artificial sweeteners in some treats can be extremely harmful to our pets. Nuts are hard for pets to digest and some, such as macadamia, can cause temporary paralysis. Just because people eat it DOES NOT mean it is safe for our cats.

Count your blessings during this season of thanks and be ever so grateful that a four-legged friend has chosen to share his life with you!!!

Christmas / Hannukah / Kwanzaa & Other Festive Celebrations

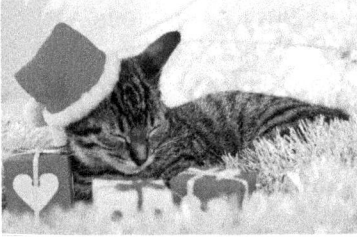

Put yourself in your cat's paws…At the end of each year, boxes are dragged from the garage or attic and unusual things happen in their home. A tree is brought INDOORS; shiny, dangly things are hung all around, and there's always food on the counter or baking in the oven while people come in and out shouting greetings!

As you decorate, whether it be electric cords, candles, pine trees or ribbon, realize any of these can be problematic and that your kitten should never be allowed to explore around them without supervision. ***Don't block pathways with decorations.*** If your cat lays on a certain window sill daily, DO NOT, DO NOT put the Christmas tree or candle display in that window!

Make sure your kitten or cat has a **safe refuge** when company comes, music gets too loud or there is any type of commotion so that they can feel safe. Also provide them with something in a quiet place to keep them out of mischief — safe toys, scratching post, kitty tree, maybe even quietly play music or a radio to drown out noise coming from the boisterous humans.

Giving pets as gifts is a very bad idea! People and families should choose the pet that is right for them, one who fits into their lifestyle and at a time they are capable of giving it a forever home. If however you have decided to adopt a cat for yourself at this time of year, that is a wonderful thing! Remember baby cats are like baby humans in that they need extra care and constant watching. They have not learned any of life's rules yet or the methods for their own survival, so…Don't upset their routine. Keep feeding and playtimes on schedule in spite of company or other obligations, and don't delay in cleaning out the litter box in spite of your extra busy schedule.

When choosing to adopt any pet during the holidays, you should consider whether or not you are willing to take a "time out" from the season. We're not saying you can't enjoy festivities because sharing them with your new best friend can be awesome, but a new pet needs time to transition into his new life and can't do so if you are dashing about, stressed, or have a constant stream of company coming and going. It's important for you to get off on the right paw and let your new furry family member know that this is now their home too and that you are their special person and will always be there for them. Remember you need to train kitty where the litter box is and what NOT to get into to keep her safe. This takes time and patience. Additionally, since the holidays are the time of year people tend to spend large quantities of money, do you have enough funds to provide your new feline friend with a proper bed, scratching post, toys, food, initial veterinary visit and emergency visit should the need arrive? If you've answered yes to all of these basic pet parenting obligations and agree to the commitment, then by all means, adopt as pets need homes for the holidays and shouldn't have to wait in a shelter a moment longer than necessary. But waiting for their soul mate person is better than being adopted into a home and lifestyle that is not ready for them. When humans get too overwhelmed, pets feel our frustration and often get returned to shelters, so make sure you are ready, and that is the best time to adopt!

Although poinsettias are the first **plants** that come to mind as a hazard around pets, they are not as dangerous as others, usually only erupting into digestive upsets. With cats, beware of Lilies! As few as two leaves/petals of certain types (stargazer, tiger, casablanca, asiatic and others) can cause kidney failure in cats. Holly, mistletoe, pine cones and pine needles can cause problems ranging from obstructions, intestinal perforations to vomiting, diarrhea and lethargy. Poisoning is relative depending on the amount of poison ingested vs. the size of the pet. See Poisonous Plant Chart on page 212. Make sure animals do not drink water from live Christmas trees as the sap, as well as any water additives, can be problematic. Cut an X in a plastic lid that will fit over the water reservoir or cover with foil. Placing "sticky tape" around your tree skirt or anything with a bumpy surface (such as an upside down floor or car mat that have those nubs cats won't like to step on) may make your pet take a step back.

Ribbons, bows, yarn and tinsel as well as cranberry and popcorn garlands on your tree or packages can entice any feline. The strings not only can cause choking and blockages but can also wrap around kitty's tongue while the other end gets pulled by intestinal contractions.

Homemade ornaments and play dough made from salt and flour can be toxic if ingested. Boxes and paper bags are generally a safe play toy for your furry friends but just be extra safe in checking these items before you toss them as kitty could be hanging out in one!

Giving kitty something to play with on the low branches may be okay, but know your kitty. If your cat can be appeased with soft ornaments, catnip toys and other safe playthings on the bottom branches, then by all means do so. But if this is only going to lead to her further exploring UP the tree, just keep her away altogether by discouraging her from hanging out by the tree — think about it…you've just provided your feline family with a great climbing perch. If they topple it, lights, breakable ornaments and cat go crashing to the floor. As a precaution, secure tree to a wall or a cup hook in the ceiling with pretty ribbon or invisible fishing wire so that at the least, it won't fall if kitty goes for a climb. Citrus smell often keeps pets at bay, so oranges, lemons and grapefruits under the tree may help. Placing a decorative child gate (think pretty white pickets) around the base may prevent your cat from getting too near and keep her safe through the season.

As for holiday eats… A little boiled or broiled white meat chicken or turkey is usually not a bad idea, although you may be surprised to learn that more and more cats have allergies to chicken and fish! The key is moderation and staying away from dark meats, cooked fats and skins, gravies and anything slathered with oils, butter or salt. If you slip a little turkey into your pet's bowl it's one thing, but remind Uncle Bob, Cousin Charlie, Grandma, your sister-in-law and the kid down the street not to also do the same. Pancreatitis can result which means your cat will need to spend the holidays in intensive care at your local Animal ER! Pets can eat fat, bone, and gristle from animals caught in the wild but once we cook fat it becomes grease; cooked bones splinter, so stick to their appropriate diet and give them safe treats. Watch out for the dropped rum balls and brandy soaked cakes as well. Cooked carrot slices, broccoli or string beans (without the salt and butter) can be a nice change; dehydrate liver or fish or make another cat treat yourself so that you know what is in it and have kitty grass available. Cats are obligate carnivores meaning they should not be vegetarians, yet even the lion in the wild eats some grass with his meal.

When keeping food hot during parties, make sure Sterno™-type canisters remain out of paws reach. They may look like pet food, and although considered "green" and clean burning, they contain ethanol and methanol which are toxic if ingested by your pet!

Don't let pets lick up spills or lick out of wine or cocktail glasses. A small amount of alcohol for a small creature can result in serious symptoms. Grapes or raisins, chocolate or caffeine products all pose dangers to our feline friends as do nuts and too much dairy (including cheeses). So supervise bowls of nuts and candies — especially if the candies are in wrappers and the cellophane too could be consumed.

Dedicate playtime just for you and your cat(s) BEFORE company arrives, and then let the kitties retreat to a quiet back bedroom with safe toys of their own to play with. Know how your cat reacts to people and noise. Welcome her to join and if you feel she can make a brief appearance, but remind children not to bother cats while they are eating and not to pull ears or tail. If kitty's ears and whiskers go back, it's time for socializing to cease. There are various interactive toys on the market to keep your cat busy while safe in a separate room, so investigate and keep her stress-free. A cat in a room full of company can easily escape out an opened door or window, so give guests a few rules about keeping kitty's home secure.

TRAVEL SAFETY

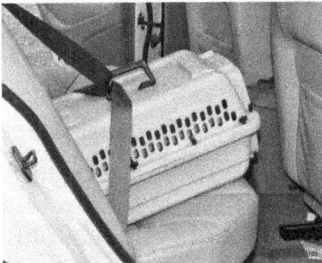

Photo Courtesy of Sunny-dog Ink.

Every year thousands of animals are injured, die or become lost in car accidents. They can be thrown against dashboards, windows, seat backs or floors.

"Wearing your seat belt costs you nothing," states Nicole Nason of the National Highway Traffic Safety Administration (NHTSA), "but the cost for not wearing one certainly will." This applies to pets too! Unrestrained pets who survive may still suffer devastating injuries. Others escape the car through broken windows and now-open doors only to end up being struck by on-coming vehicles.

Cause of Accidents
Pets are often the cause of accidents. According to the American Automobile Association (AAA), animals moving around in cars are the third worst distraction to a driver ranking only behind children and cell phones.

Ways to Keep Your Cat Safe
No excuses! Kitty crates, carriers and travel seats are also good choices as they shield pets from falling objects. Just make sure the crate too is secured so that it along with your cat or dog does not become a projectile during an impact or sudden stop.

Do not Let Your Cat Ride "Shotgun"

If the airbag is deployed it could crush your cat or break her neck. Airbags have been known to shatter fiberglass carriers so kitty is better off in her crate in the back seat with it firmly secured inside the car!

Several campaigns have been launched to help you become proactive for the safety of your pet, and new products become available all the time, so become a savvy pet parent keeping your eyes open for new ways to keep your best friend safe.

When going out of town, have your cat examined by your Veterinarian and make sure vaccinations are current. Next, get your cat acclimated to the car by taking short trips close to home. Should your traveling companion need a bit of calming, CDs are available that can relax the whole family en route as can Rescue Remedy® to spritz anxiety away. An inside-the-carrier litter box is a must and NEVER leave your cat alone in the car for even a few minutes. Despite windows rolled down, cars get very hot very fast and your best friend could suffer brain damage.

Choosing Your Mode of Transportation

TIPS FOR DECREASING MOTION SICKNESS:

1) Allow your kitty to spend good quality time in the car with you without the engine running and give him positive reinforcement for good behavior.
2) Follow this up with short trips around the block slowly providing ear scratches and treats at your destination.

NOTE: A few bites of a ginger snap cookie 20 minutes before any car ride often settles some queasy feline tummies. If using pure ginger capsules, give 150 mg per 10 lbs. of body weight 30 minutes before departure and repeat every 8 hours.

3) As you increase road travel, always make sure it is on an empty stomach – that your pet has not eaten for 4-6 hours.
4) Confining your cat not only makes safety sense, but it restricts her movement lessening the likelihood of nausea. If your cat is riding in a crate or carrier, facing the crate forward helps prevent motion sickness. If you must turn it in another direction for safety sake, cover it to prevent your cat looking out in a non-forward moving direction. For safely restraining a cat while traveling (see page 74).
5) If you have more than one vehicle, try them out with Fluffy. Some cars vibrate more or are more conducive to motion sickness than others.
6) Keep the car cool inside.
7) If motion sickness seems to be an ongoing problem for your cat, speak to your Veterinarian about Cerenia (maropitant citrate) or other prescription medications that won't make your kitty drowsy but will allow her to spend her time on four wheels with you. As with all drugs, follow directions to the letter for your cat's sake.
8) If the problem seems more anxiety related, aromatherapy with lavender may prove beneficial in keeping nerves at bay.

Planes

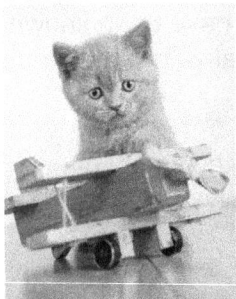

If you need to get there fast, a plane may be your choice of transport. Check with the various commercial carriers for their rules and regulations to see which can best accommodate your cat on board. Air Hollywood's K9 Flight School prepares people and pets to travel confidently and comfortably by providing valuable information and training in an immersive aviation environment. It might be good to give this a try before leaving on the real thing!

Here are some considerations to increase the chances of a safe flight:

- Familiarize your cat with her travel carrier weeks before the flight and don't forget a pre-travel veterinary visit.
- Clip nails so that they can't catch on carrier doors, and make sure the collar also cannot catch on anything.
- Don't feed for 4-6 hours prior to air travel. Place ice cubes in the tray attached to the inside of the crate. Water will spill.
- Once through security it will be hours before a potty break, Check if a disposable litter pan would be allowed in the carrier, inside the cabin.
- Book only direct flights and chose early morning/late evening flights during the hot months and afternoon flights during the colder times of year. Avoid holiday chaos at all costs for your pet's sake.
- Let the captain and flight attendants know your pet is traveling with you.
- Label the carrier with your name, permanent address and telephone number, final destination, and where you or a contact person can be reached as soon as the flight arrives.
- Upon arrival, open the carrier as soon as you are in a safe place and if anything appears not quite right, high tail it to a Veterinarian.

Trains

Traveling by train may be considered a cultural experience, but felines don't get it, and the noise and vibration may be a stressful experience. Most animals must ride in cargo without climate controls, so consider the time of year and all the usual travel precautions such as ID-ing your cat, acclimating her ahead of time, how frequently you can visit with her and everything else you can think of to make her journey stress-free.

Must-Haves for the Traveling Feline: Your Pet's Travel Kit

No matter where you go, there are items Fluffy should not be without:

- Health certificate/vaccination records in duplicate
- Medications and supplements (flea & tick prevention)
- Bowls (food and water)
- Usual food (don't chance a stomach upset by switching on the road)
- Water (in the car and plane, ice cubes work best when available)
- Treats and/or Meal Replacement Bars
- Micro-chip and ID tag on a securely fitting collar
- Extra leashes, harness, travel seat/carrier
- Cat First-Aid Kit and handbook
- Ginger snaps to settle an upset tummy. Rescue Remedy® for anxiety.
- Canned or dehydrated pumpkin puree (no added ingredients unless plain apple fiber) for most kinds of digestive upsets (vomiting, diarrhea and constipation)
- Information regarding Veterinarians and 24 Hour Pet Emergency Hospitals (a great resource is "Pet E.R. Guide" by Melinda Lord, Trailer Life Books but also check for up-to-date Apps)
- Bedding and something that smells like home
- Toys
- Crate
- Brush & towels
- Lint brushes or packaging tape so you don't leave too much hair wherever you go
- Kitty sweater if temperature drops

Pet Travel Expert Janine Franceschi says , "The most important item I carry when Beau and I travel together is a complete copy of all of his medical records. You hope you never need them, but when you do it makes life so much easier to have them handy than trying to get in touch with a vet thousands of miles away."

Debra Jo Chiapuzio recommends that you also "bring along knowledge and peace of mind by knowing what to do in an emergency situation – learn pet first-aid and CPR." See Section II of this book to get yourself up-to-speed on these skills.

Disaster Preparedness

Do your research now and gather your tools, so that if an emergency occurs, you can turn tragedy into a success story for your four-legged family members.

Hopefully you will never experience a fire destroying your home, yet you plan ahead -- install fire alarms, smoke detectors and purchase insurance. You certainly hope never to be involved in a car accident, but you have airbags and wear a seat belt (and should safely restrain your cat as well). Being prepared makes sense as we can minimize potential injury to those we love. However, most people are not prepared for a major disaster. "Be Prepared" works for the Scouts, and it's a motto we should carry into our adult lives. Planning ahead is the best way to keep yourself and your cat safe.

At The Very Least:

Photo: Sunny-dog Ink

1) Place a Pet Alert Sticker near you front door recording how many and what type of animals live there. If you aren't home when tragedy strikes, trained professionals will seek out and help your pets.

2) Designate a pre-arranged meeting place for your family and identify several places that can take your pets. Red Cross Shelters do not permit pets. Many organizations train communities to set-up temporary animal shelters, but it could still be days before these facilities are in place. Making arrangements ahead of time with out-of-town friends and relatives is your best bet, but have a "Plan B." Susan Keyes, President of the Southern California Animal Response Team says, "Long-term housing and care for pets is the area we have found people to be least prepared." Check with pet day care and boarding facilities as well as your Veterinarian to see if they will accommodate during a disaster. Compile a list of hotels where pets are welcome and set aside one credit card just for emergency use. It's also a good idea to have cash (in bills smaller than 20s) easily accessible as ATM Machines will not be working.

Know pet-friendly locations before you need them. Publisher Susan Sims and her team at "Fido Friendly" are a great place to start your research.

3) Stash the following for each pet in an easy-to-carry backpack or crate (that way you'll have the carrier to evacuate in):
   - A two-week supply of food stored in an airtight container and a manual can opener if needed; water; medication. Remember to exchange these items regularly so they are fresh when needed.
   - A water-proof container with vaccination & micro-chipping records and photos of your cat with your family as proof of ownership.
   - Treats, toys, bedding, food & water dishes; collars/harnesses and leashes; litter, scoop & boxes; disinfectant for cleaning crates, paper towels, flashlight with batteries, zip ties, garbage bags and a well-stocked Cat First-Aid Kit.

4) Stay Informed by listening to media announcements for frequent updates. As the saying goes, "Knowledge is power," so don't be caught unaware.

See checklist on page 206.

Where To Put It All
Even with the best laid plans, life happens, so consider storing your goods in several locations in the event they are un-retrievable when the ground shakes, the flames rise or the mud slides. Positioning items close to an outside wall in your home will allow easier access should buildings collapse and you need to rummage through rubble to get to your supplies. Also, stowing duplicate items in your car is a good idea.

Don't Forget The Two-Legged Family Members
Also remember to keep a stash of food and other items for the humans including a battery or solar-powered radio, rubber-soled shoes and a flashlight near your bed so that you can help your pets and stay safe!

Determine well in advance which rooms are safest should you need to hunker down (center of house, bathrooms, closets, basements, or other room depending on type of impending danger.)

In situations where water supply may become contaminated, fill up bathtubs and sinks to ensure that you have access to water during a power outage or other crises.

Preparing for the worst may just prevent the worst from happening!

Tips for Specific Disasters
Although it is difficult to teach someone not to get stressed, being as prepared as you can be for any situation in life can help lessen the panic that sets in when the worst happens. Follow general disaster preparedness Tips, but also take special care depending on which of the following natural disasters are likely to occur in your part of the world.

Hurricanes
The one good thing to be said about hurricanes is that they are predictable -- The National Hurricane Center tracks weather patterns and notes possible disturbances long before they pose a threat. It's imperative that you monitor your local news channels and once a Hurricane Watch is issued, although you may have 24 - 36 hours before it hits, don't wait to do the following:

- Keep pets indoors and easily accessible should you need to suddenly pack them up and leave. Cats can sense impending doom and often hide, so get them into a carrier early.
- Stay tuned to news stations for evacuation routes and make sure you completely understand the plan.
- Have at least one week's food, water and any medications stored for your pets and prep your house for the storm (board-up windows, stow away items that can blow such as patio furniture, secure gates, etc.).

A Hurricane Warning is issued when the storm is 24 hours away or less. Complete all preparations before the rain and high winds arrive, and stay in your home only if it is safe. If you evacuate, take your cat with you.

Wildfires

Once underway, wildfires can consume millions of acres and blow in changing directions. For this reason, you should plan several escape routes for you and your pets in the event the flames block your path.

- Create a "fire break" around your home by clearing away vegetation, especially dead brush, about 30 feet from all structures.
- Use fabric, rope or leather leashes and collars. Nylon ones melt when heated and can badly burn your pet.
- Take all animals with you. Monitor your pets for burns and smoke inhalation. Knowing how to perform Rescue Breathing & CPR could save your cat's life!

Earthquakes

Unlike most natural disasters, there is no advanced warning for an earthquake allowing no time for last minute precautions. In addition to covering the steps above:

- Never position catios, crates or enclosures underneath objects that could fall during a tremor.
- Add a pair of bolt cutters to your disaster kit in case damaged cages or fencing need opening.
- Know where to turn off the gas to your house, barn or kennels.
- Include your pets in the family earthquake drill and make sure all family members know how to handle them realizing that a frightened pet may bite or scratch.
- If you board your pet, make sure the facility knows of your earthquake preparedness plans.

Should an earthquake occur, confine your cats. Pets that escape sometimes return at mealtime, but there are no guarantees! Be prepared to handle cut and burned paws, know how to splint broken bones and stop bleeding in humans and animals alike. In other words, take a Cat First-Aid Class before you wish you had.

Floods

Floods can affect any part of the world and can even be confined to only your home or apartment building. Every year hundreds of thousands of people are forced to evacuate due to rising water. Slowly rising water is usually due to rivers, streams or even a pipe leak in your home. Flash floods however can hit quickly caused by heavy rain or melting snow as well as failure to a dam or reservoir.

- Map out several evacuation routes for yourself and your four-legged family; don't rely on only one which may be in the path of the floodwater. Head for the nearest high ground with your pets, and it is always better to err on the side of caution and evacuate early. If it is a false alarm, you and your family have practiced a meaningful drill instead of the real thing.

- Never leave any animal behind and certainly don't tie up an animal if flood waters threaten. You cannot anticipate how high water may rise, so even birds enclosed on high perches could perish.
- Remember that danger of disease can be an issue after a flood. Keep pets away from standing water. Have a good fresh supply of water on hand for everyone (1/2 gallon per day for cats) as even tap water may not be safe if contaminated water has entered the drinking supply.

Make Your Older Pet's Years Golden

With the ceremonial lighting of candle #7 on the cat's birthday cake, it is generally assumed your best friend has embarked on her golden years. Though often premature to consider her a senior citizen, it's a great time to make changes that can ensure a continuing quality of life. Decreased activity and loss of muscle tone can result in constipation, arthritis, degenerative joint disease and cognitive dysfunction, so get those paws moving. But always speak with your Veterinarian before starting any new regimen to be sure it is the best course of action for your cat and bring her in for a senior wellness exam.

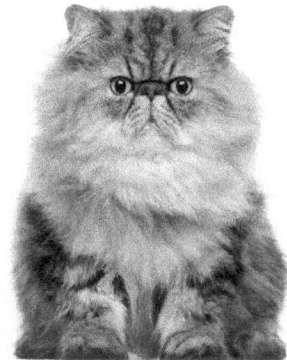

Felines and humans experience many of the same aging patterns: graying hair, aches, pains and stiffness, sleeping more and slowing down. One big difference though is that our cats can't tell us what hurts or what isn't working as good as it used to. Your Veterinarian can be a great source in determining your pet's needs, but you are even better. Pay attention, really get to know your cat and observe any changes to insure her later years will be truly golden.

Exercise helps maintain healthy body weight -
Just as in humans, excess weight in senior pets may bring about serious health conditions. Without proper exercise, the increased bulk stresses an older cat's heart. When this organ doesn't function properly, other organs like the brain, lungs, liver and kidneys suffer too. Exercise also aids in proper digestion and nutrient absorption which are important to overall health.

Exercise helps delay the onset of osteoarthritis – We all need our joints to work smoothly and efficiently to get us where we want to go. Moderate exercise can keep movement fluid, slow deterioration and minimize pain.

Exercise helps maintain mental health – Well-oxygenated blood flow to tissues does a body good, and exercise also removes toxins. Activity keeps nutrients like glucose at optimum levels in the brain and like every other organ in the body, the brain requires good nutrition to function properly.

Quality time with and loving touch from you – It has been discovered that human touch can stimulate parts of the brain that control emotions in human Alzheimer patients so why not give it a try with your furry best friend?

What's a cat parent to do?

- First, talk to your Veterinarian to determine what exercises will be most beneficial and which to avoid.
- If at any time your cat appears tired, coughs or has problems breathing, stop and call your vet. You know your cat better than anyone else and know when she is not acting normal. By detecting and treating a problem early, you may save your best friend's life.
- Remain patient with your older cat and never get frustrated with her changing behaviors and attitudes. Enjoy each moment together.
- Don't over-treat during training as older cats add weight more quickly and lose pounds more slowly due to changes in their metabolism.

Whatever you do, do it together and cherish those golden years!

A Few PAWSitive Actions to Keep Your Senior Cat Comfy

1) Felines and humans experience many of the same aging patterns -- graying hair, aches, pains and stiffness, sleeping more and slowing down. One big difference though is that our ***cats can't (and probably wouldn't if they could) tell us what hurts or what isn't working as good as it used to.*** Your veterinarian can be a great source in determining your cat's needs, but you are even better. Pay attention, really get to know your cat and observe any changes to insure his later years will be truly golden.

2) As animals age, ***they often can't "hold it,"*** and need more frequent bathroom breaks. Other times they have trouble remembering to ask to go out. **Don't lose patience** with your loyal companion. Cats can benefit from a second litter box being added to the household to allow them time to reach their "bathroom." Especially if you live in a split-level home, having an upstairs and a downstairs kitty latrine can really make life easier for your older feline. Make sure also that the box isn't difficult for older bones to crawl into.

3) All pets should have ***a special place of their own***, but senior cats should have **a bed in a draft- free, damp-free location** – something they can easily get out of but that cushions their aching joints. Observe your kitty for her choice of location; some like the comfort of an egg-crate mattress while others prefer the coolness of the floor.

   Cats love sunning themselves, but as they age, the jump up to the windowsill may be a chore. Place a chair or bench under the window so that Fluffy can still enjoy her favorite spot without the pain or fear of having to make the leap.

4) **<u>Supplements</u>** - Talk with your veterinarian or holistic practitioner about other supplements that could help maintain healthy tendons, ligaments, joints and cartilage such as: Glucosamine Sulfate with MSM, Chondroitin, Hyaluronic Acid and others. Other supplements may positively impact your pet's lifestyle including CBD, PCR Hemp Oil, Vitamin E, Melatonin, Essential Fatty Acids and Curcumin for example, but check with your pet's medical professional. Don't just add these items to your pet's diet without knowing how they might react with other medications or treatments.

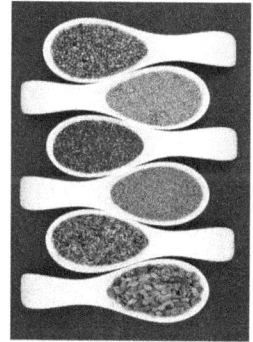

5) A cat with (or without) hearing loss must be protected by being ***<u>kept safely indoors!</u>***. As senses dim, your pet won't hear approaching traffic, children or other animals coming near. When startled he may snap or bite out of fear. Be aware of changes. Teach everyone to gently stomp their feet to ***<u>create a vibration</u>*** your pet can feel and call out when approaching a hearing or vision impaired pet. **<u>Use hand signals</u>** when your voice can no longer be heard; flick kitchen lights to teach your deaf pet that it's time for dinner.

6) ***<u>Don't rearrange the furniture!</u>*** Pets with fading sight memorize their pathways. Keep them safe by installing a gate near stairs so that they can't take a tumble, and build a wide, sturdy ramp over steps your dog frequents.

7) ***<u>Various modalities</u>*** such as chiropractic adjustments, massage (see page 24), stretching, aquatic therapy and acupuncture can make a world of difference in the mobility of some senior cats.

8) ***<u>Make time</u>*** for ear scratches or whatever your kitty likes best. Senior cats do best when they know they are loved......short walks, car rides or just being together. Senior pets do best when they know they are loved and are still a treasured part of the family.

End of Life Decisions

The loss of a beloved pet can be devastating as our cats are part of our family.
As your cat gets on in years or develops a chronic condition, talk with the family about what is best for your best friend. Although wonderful advances have been made in feline medicine, putting your pet through surgery and extensive medication may not provide them the best quality of life for their golden years. Although we selfishly may not want to say good bye, euthanasia administered by a caring veterinarian with your family present may be the kindest last gift you can give your pet. Investigate professionals who come to your home to make that transition easier as well as offer tips on how to make those last days, weeks and months memorable for all.

Before the time comes, decide on a pet cemetery or having your cat cremated. Most cities do not allow burying of pets in your backyard, so research ahead so you won't hit road blocks while you are grieving.

And all family members must take time to grieve. Some may benefit from talking to like-minded people who understand. Veterinary colleges have hotlines manned by students trained in grief counseling.

Help your child (and yourself) cope by encouraging them to talk about how much they miss their friend. Look at photographs of happy times with your kitty and help your child plan a goodbye ceremony for their special friend. Well-meaning euphemisms like the cat "went to sleep" may worry some children about going to bed fearing they too may not wake up. Speak in clear yet simple terms.

Do pets grieve? You bet they do! Give your other best-friends time and grieve along with them. Increase your bond by spending quality time together. Just like us, working through grief takes time and every pet exhibits different behaviors. Some may sleep near the deceased pet's bed, toys or food dishes and appear sad while others may act as if nothing has changed. When the time is right, loving another canine or feline family member can help heal the heart but never replaces the old friend you said goodbye to.

Every cat will leave their own unique set of paw prints on your heart!

The Rainbow Bridge
Author Unknown but inspired by a Norse Legend

By the edge of a woods, at the foot of a hill,
Is a lush, green meadow where time stands still.
Where the friends of man and woman do run,
When their time on earth is over and done.
For here, between this world and the next,
Is a place where each beloved creature finds rest.
On this golden land, they wait and they play,
Till the Rainbow Bridge they cross over one day.
No more do they suffer, in pain or in sadness,
For here they are whole, their lives filled with gladness.
Their limbs are restored, their health renewed,
Their bodies have healed, with strength imbued.
They romp through the grass, without even a care,
Until one day they start, and sniff at the air.
All ears prick forward, eyes dart front and back,
Then all of a sudden, one breaks from the pack.
For just at that instant, their eyes have met;
Together again, both person and pet.
So they run to each other, these friends from long past,
The time of their parting is over at last.
The sadness they felt while they were apart,
Has turned into joy once more in each heart.
They embrace with a love that will last forever,
And then, side-by-side, they cross over… together.

Why You Should Know Pet First-Aid and CPR

Without warning, tragedy can strike, so you must know what to do when something happens. Have you ever driven down a dimly lit road to narrowly escape hitting an animal? Has an outdoor cookout ever tempted your feline to claw at a sizzling treat? Has a furry tail ever been accidentally closed in a door, or have you found ticks on your long-haired cat? Did you discover a cat in a car suffering from heat stroke this summer? How about vomiting, diarrhea and bee stings – have your pets ever experienced these problems? Statistics show that preventable accidents are the leading cause of death among our pets, and 9 out of 10 dogs and cats can expect to have an emergency during their lifetime. *According to the American Animal Hospital Association (AAHA), one out of four additional animals could be saved if just one Pet First-Aid technique was applied prior to the animal receiving veterinary care.* What this means is that the most competent Veterinarian cannot bring your pet back to life, but by knowing Pet First-Aid & CPR, you can keep your cat alive until you reach professional medical help.

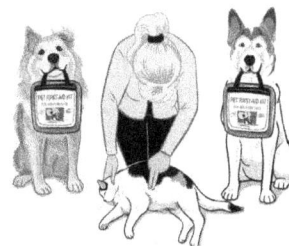

Although Veterinarians are the experts, they are generally not on the scene when something happens to your pet, so it is up to YOU to react quickly and effectively before professional medical care is available. Knowing what to do during those first few moments can truly make a difference for your feline. What this means is that if you know how to stop bleeding and how to bandage a wound, you can prevent your cat from great blood loss and keep infection at bay; if you can reduce your cat's body temperature, you can prevent brain damage and death, and if you can alleviate choking, you can stop your cat from going unconscious. Cat First-Aid is not a replacement for veterinary care. Together you and your Veterinarian should work as a team for the well-being of your cat.

How Cat First-Aid Differs From Human First-Aid

Instincts are great, if we listen to them, but very often since we're dealing with a species unlike our own, humans do the wrong thing or do nothing at all. Even if you have taken a human first-aid course, getting pet-specific training is essential since we do not share anatomies with our feline friends. The concept is the same in many instances, but the technique often differs. When giving rescue breathing to a person, we pinch off the nose and breathe into their mouth. It's the complete opposite for our cats with us closing their mouth and breathing into their nostrils. How about compressing your kitty's heart…did you realize that you must squeeze not only the rib cage but also compress the two balloons (aka the lungs) that surround the heart in order to effectively perform CPR? Since we can't ask our pets, "Where does it hurt?" or "What did you eat?", we need to constantly look for signs and symptoms of illness, and that requires us to tune in and really get to know our pets as well as learn the correct protocols.

Another big difference between human and animal patients is that animals might bite out of fear or pain. You must at all times be aware of your pet's changing body language so that an animal injury does not turn into a human first aid incident. You must know how to appropriately restrain and handle an injured animal and check the scene for any hazards before you begin tending to your precious cat because if you get injured, you will be unable to care for the injured animal. Furthermore, animals that are known to have bitten a person – even if the bite occurred during an emergency situation in which the animal was in pain – will require quarantine until rabies has been ruled out. Therefore, pet-specific training is essential for your pet's sake and yours as well.

Refer To Pet Safety Page 30 For Animal Body Language

By Knowing Cat First-Aid You Can:

- Lower your cat's body temperature if he suffers from heat stroke and prevent brain damage or death.

- Stop bleeding and prevent infection by properly bandaging a wound.

- Prevent your cat from losing consciousness by alleviating choking.

- Expel poison from your cat's system by properly inducing vomiting.

- Be the pump your cat's heart can't be until you can get her to professional medical help.

- By learning what can happen to your cat, you may prevent many emergencies from ever happening.

CAT FIRST-AID FOR INJURIES AND ILLNESSES

What is Cat First-Aid?

Cat First-Aid is the first thing YOU do to help a cat who is ill or has been injured. It is often the most critical step as it may dictate the eventual outcome. The goal is to make the animal more comfortable, lower the risk of infection and stop further injury before complete medical attention can be given.

In certain scenarios, after performing first-aid, you may just need to observe your kitty until she heals, however, first-aid is considered the MOST critical step because in worse case situations, if your cat is not breathing or does not have a pulse, she could die before you get her in the car and to your Veterinarian's office. By knowing how to administer CPCR, YOU, can keep your cat alive until you reach your animal emergency center. If you don't jump to action at the time the emergency occurs, veterinary professionals may not be able to use their expertise to save your pet, for if she has expired…no medicine or surgery will bring them back.

Additionally, if you apply even one Pet First-Aid technique, you may limit your cat's pain and time to heal and even save money. By controlling blood loss, you may avoid the need for transfusions. By limiting an injured cat's movements, you can prevent further damage to a limb which could result in a longer recuperative period and additional pain. These and many other reasons you will discover in this book (and in the course of being a pet lover) make it imperative that you learn Cat First-Aid. It is crucial for the health and safety of your cat and may allow her to live a longer life with you!

Finally, in every first-aid situation, be prepared to treat for "shock," so hone up on those skills on page 188.

Types of Emergency Situations: ABCs = Airway, Breathing, Circulation

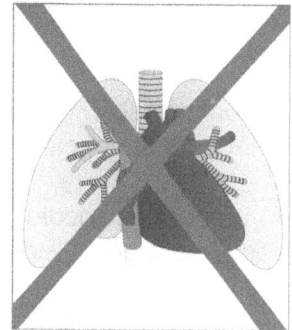

No matter if it's a dog, cat or human, these are the only three scenarios you will encounter:

1) **Heart & lungs are working but something is not right.** Distress may range from mild digestive upset to unconsciousness, choking, bleeding, seizures, etc. Depending upon the type of distress, this may or may not be a life-threatening situation.

> You need to perform: **Cat First-Aid** (the type of distress will determine the type of first–aid administered.)

2) **Lungs have stopped.** Heart is working (a pulse can be detected), but the lungs have stopped functioning. The absence of breathing should be considered a life-threatening emergency. Always check for breathing first. The rule is that if the animal is breathing, the heart is beating.

> You need to perform: **Rescue Breathing**

3) **Heart and lungs have both stopped.** No pulse can be detected and the animal has stopped breathing. Within a matter of minutes, irreparable cell damage will occur. This is always considered a life-threatening emergency.

> You must begin: **CPCR** -- Cardio Pulmonary Cerebral Resuscitation (Commonly referred to as CPR.)

Work as a Team With Your Veterinarian

How To Select Your Veterinarian

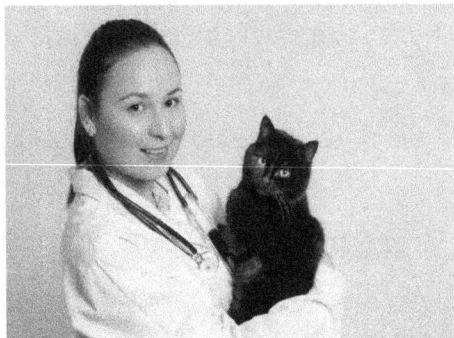

In addition to checking out your prospective Veterinarian's qualifications, make sure that he or she is someone that you feel you can talk freely with about your pet's condition and receive answers that are easily understood. Consider the expertise and experience with issues and conditions that your pet may experience. Take in to account your Veterinarian's inclination to consider a variety of treatment options and the Veterinarian's willingness to research and explain those in a manner that you can understand and feel comfortable with. Your Veterinarian should have a general concern for your pet's well-being and their office should not be so busy that it takes days to get an appointment.

A Veterinarian should not only be competent regarding your cat's care, but they should also have a good bedside manner toward your four-legged family member. Ask around and listen to what other pet parents have to say. Check if your Veterinarian is a Fear Free® Certified and a member of member of the American Animal Hospital Association (AAHA) and if the office is also AAHA Certified. Consider the obvious when visiting your pet's medical doctor. Is the office clean? Are there separate areas for dogs and cats so that your timid cat won't be subjected to a room full of barking dogs? Is the front office staff helpful, attentive and friendly and do they remain at the facility year after year? Sometimes when the front office team changes frequently, it signals that something is not quite right at the business.

Remember that your Veterinarian is your pet's SECOND Best Friend (you, of course are number one) and plays a vital role as a key member in your pet's health team. Also see pages 7 - 10 for your Cat's Health & Safety Team.

Locate Your Nearest Animal Emergency Center

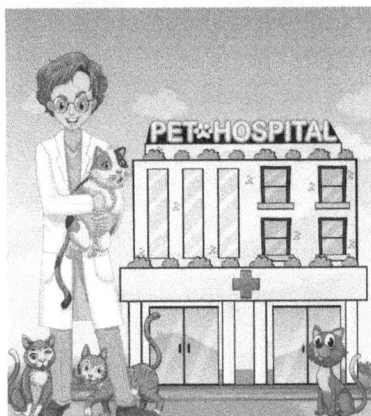

Some are open 24 hours; others open at 6pm and close at 8am the next morning to fill that gap of time when your Veterinarian is closed. Locate the one nearest your home, and wherever you and your pet spend time. Make sure you know exactly where the office is located, where to park and what entrance you will bring your pet in. Know what services they offer (MRIs, transfusions, antivenin, ambulance transport) and how they accept payment. Research all this ahead of time because when an emergency happens, time can mean the difference between life and death for your cat.

Needless worrying about which side of the street the Animal ER is on or what services they provide can be avoided by doing your homework. Being prepared applies to cat parents too and could save you time as well as your cat's life.

Fill in your important info in the back of this book on page 206 so that you have contact info at your fingertips when needed.

Most Common Situations That ALWAYS Require Veterinary Care

Regardless of what first-aid techniques you perform to alleviate pain and make your pet more comfortable, for the injuries below you MUST seek immediate veterinary care.

This list is by no means all-inclusive of situations requiring veterinary assistance, so if in doubt, always seek the advice of a licensed Veterinarian. Rather this list lets you know that if you have a cat experiencing any of these ailments, get him to your Veterinarian immediately! Details will be provided on pages to come as to how you can provide first-aid care to animals for the situations listed below.

1) Anytime you have administered rescue breathing or CPR (even if your kitty seems okay afterwards) or if the pet is having any difficulty breathing
2) Trauma to the head, chest or abdomen or anytime an animal has been unconscious
3) First-time seizure, seizure lasting more than five minutes, or in cases of an epileptic animal, a seizure lasting longer than is normal for that pet
4) Arterial or venous bleeding (major blood loss)
5) Fractures or suspected muscle/tendon strains or tears
6) Wounds more than 1" in length and/or more than ½" deep including bites and especially those which are prone to abscesses and infections
7) Suspected or known poisoning or snake bites
8) Shock (depletion of oxygen to the body due to blood loss, trauma, anaphylaxis or pulmonary/cardiac arrest -- a life-threatening condition you will learn more about in this book)
9) Inability to walk
10) Unconscious

For any of the above, do immediate first-aid and then...

GET TO YOUR Veterinarian AT ONCE!

Assessing Your Cat's Health

Learning to check your pet's vitals can help assess his degree of pain, injury or illness.

There are 5 vital checks that you should be able to perform.

The 5 Vital Checks:

1) **Pulse** – The rhythmic movement of blood through an artery.
   - Place the ball of two fingers (not your thumb) on the depression found in the kitty's upper inner thigh over the femoral artery.
   - Count the beats for 60 seconds (or for 30 seconds and then multiply by 2 to determine pulse rate.)
   - Take the pulse over 3-5 days to determine the baseline number for your pet.

If you have difficulty feeling the femoral artery, place the palm of your hand over the left side of the chest – just behind her elbow – to feel heart beat which will be the same rate.

Average Heart Rate For Cats	
Species	**Average Heart Rate**
Cats	160 - 200 Beats Per Minute

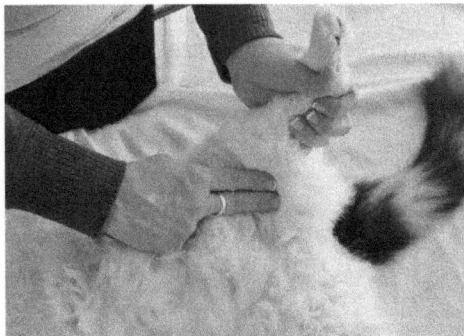

Photo by Sunny-dog Ink

2) Respiration – The process of inhaling and exhaling; breathing.

- Observe or place your hand over the cat's chest to count the number of times her chest rises (inhales) or falls (exhales). The "rise and fall cycle" should be counted as one breath.
- Count the breaths (rise and fall cycles) for 60 seconds (or for 30 seconds and then multiply by 2) to determine respirations per minute.
- Check respiration over 3-5 days on your cat to determine the baseline number.
- Do not attempt to count the respirations of a panting cat.

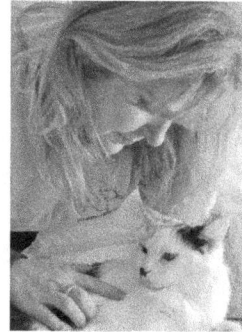

Average Heart & Respiration Rate For Cats	
Species	**Average Heart & Respiration Rate**
Cats	20 - 40 Breaths Per Minute

Please Note: *Very large cats and geriatric animals may have slower respirations. Rule of thumb is that the bigger and older the cat, the slower their pulse or respiraton. The smaller and younger the cat, the faster their breathing and pulse rate.*

3) Temperature – The level of heat produced by the body.

- After lubricating the tip of a digital thermometer with petroleum jelly or other such safe product, lift cat's tail up to access the area and prevent them from sitting, and insert non-glass digital thermometer ½" – 1" into the rectum (slightly angled upward).
- At the sound of the beep or according to specific instrument instructions, the animal's temperature should range between 100.4° F – 102.5° F (38° C – 39.16° C). A temperature of 101°F is considered average cats.
- A temperature of 103° F is considered a fever.
- A temperature of 104° F and above is considered an emergency.

NOTE: Feeling your cat's nose to determine their temperature or state of health is not an accurate measurement.

4) Capillary Refill Time (CRT) -

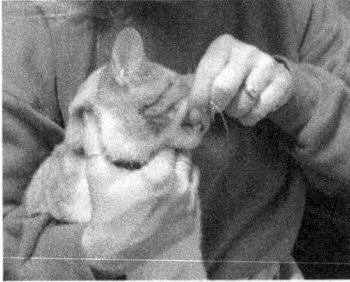

The amount of time it takes for blood and oxygen to refill a capillary (smallest vessels transporting blood and oxygen throughout the body) after pressure has been applied and released.

CRT indicates whether blood circulation is sufficient to sustain life. Sometimes referred to as perfusion.

Photo by Sunny-dog Ink

- Gently lift cat's upper lip at the side and press on gums above teeth with the ball of your index finger until gums lighten. Be sure not to pull too tight because this can cause the gums to appear lighter and make it much more difficult to accurately assess CRT.
- It is best to choose a non-pigmented part of the animal's gums if at all possible, but if you only have dark gums to work with, you should still be able to determine CRT. If you feel unsure on a dark-gummed cat, gently pull down on an eyelid to see if the inside color is pink. If it is pale, seek immediate veterinary assistance.
- Release pressure and color should return to the gums within 1-2 seconds.
- If it takes color (blood flow) longer than 2 seconds to return to gums after you have released the pressure applied by your finger, increase circulation by slightly elevating the cat's hind quarters with a pillow (unless there is significant bleeding to head or chest) and get immediate veterinary help. Also see shock on page 188.

5) Hydration – Sufficient water in an animal's body to sustain health. Dehydration is the loss of water and vital electrolytes such as sodium, chloride and potassium necessary for survival. The bodies of our feline friends are comprised of 70% to 80% water. As a reference, a 50 pound animal requires about 5 cups (or 40 ounces) of water daily, but if he's active that amount should be at least doubled. Cats are resilient and can survive the loss of up to 50% of their muscle and fat, but a dehydration level of more than 10% is life threatening.

To determine adequate hydration levels, use the following procedure:
- Gently pinch a fold of skin at animal's nape of neck and release. The skin should quickly fall back into place if animal is well hydrated. This is often referred to as the Tugor Test.
- For loose-skinned kitties and older pets whose skin may have lost elasticity, carefully feel the gums. If they are dry or sticky, the pet may be dehydrated.
- Fatigue, constipation, increased heart rate and sunken eyes can also signal dehydration.

See page 215 for a chart to fill in with YOUR pet's vitals!

Head-to-Tail Examination

In addition to checking a cat's vital statistics, it is important to observe her body for signs of injury or illness. The more you know what is normal for any cat, the more quickly you will recognize something that is not.

Start at the head and work your way toward the tail, observing the skin and coat, feeling for lumps, bumps, abrasions and parasites. Notice any red or tender areas by also paying attention to your pet's facial expressions, movements and sounds. Cats will immediately let you know that they are not amused!

Gently clean **ears** of dirt and waxy debris with appropriate ear wash and a soft cloth -- do not plunge a cotton swab into your cat's ear canal as you could cause deafness or damage. If you discover redness, parasites or a foul odor coming from your cat's ears at any time, have your Veterinarian assess at once. What may look like coffee grounds could be dirt left behind by parasites such as fleas or mites.

New products appear on the market regularly, so check with your Veterinarian as to which ones are best to use on your pet. Remember however to always follow directions closely - only use cat products for cats, and stick to the recommended doses according to body weight or other specifications. A small error could prove dangerous to your best friend. Also, watch them carefully when trying new products and observe your cat's reaction to the treatment.

If eyes tear excessively or you notice a discharge, flush with eye wash (saline solution or purified water should be the only ingredient listed).

Compare one eye to the other for any differences making sure both pupils are the same size. Cats have elliptical pupils (vertical slits), but both should respond to light by contracting and then dilating (or enlarging) when light source is removed. If pupils are not of equal size, your pet could have a condition and should be checked by a Veterinarian immediately.

Track your cat's eye movement by holding an index finger in front of his face and slowly moving it from side to side. Do her eyes follow your movements? If you detect any erratic flickers or jumps in the eyes, it could also indicate a neurological issue which a Veterinarian should assess.

Feel the **muzzle** for bumps and tenderness. Due to bone and cartilage, it may be impossible to feel a tumor, so if the area appears sore or if there is an unusual discharge from the nostrils, get to your Veterinarian for a thorough exam. Soreness on the muzzle, however, could also be coming from the mouth.

Do you brush your kitty's teeth regularly? It only takes 48 hours for plaque to turn to tartar leading to gum disease. *Carefully look in the mouth*. Gums should be a healthy pink (unless your cat has black gums) with no bad odor. Check for broken teeth and obvious signs of swelling or bleeding. Anything that doesn't appear normal should be evaluated by a Veterinarian. Cats are notorious for eating dental floss, string and tinsel which can wrap around teeth or the base of the tongue. Foreign objects that become stuck in the mouth should always be checked by your Veterinarian as they can cause inflammation or damage to the oral tissues. If your pet is suddenly losing weight or not eating, dental issues could be the cause.

The rest of your head-to-tail examination should be a gentle massage along the cat's sides and back, looking and feeling for ANYTHING that does not belong -- abrasions, bumps, tenderness and sores; even parasites, burrs and foxtails that may have found their way onto your friend's furry coat. When you reach your cat's **chest**, you should be able to feel, but not see, the ribs. Breathing should be steady. It is important that you learn to check respiration and all of your animal's vital signs so you know you are doing your best for the health of your companion. See page 215 in this book.

Inspect legs and paws making sure claws and pads are not cracked, and keep nails trimmed so that they won't catch in carpet or break on concrete let alone scratch you or your pet. Be gentle and go a speed that is comfortable for your best friend. Many animals get uneasy when touched, but examine a little at a time, and they'll come to enjoy this bonding experience.

With your fingertips, stroke the **abdomen** making sure there are no hard spots or sensitive areas. Check nipples (males have these too), genitals and "under the tail" which should all be clean with no colored discharge. If your pet is older or arthritic and can't keep up with her own daily hygiene, help keep her clean with a warm wet cloth. If you notice scooting or excessive licking, the anal glands may need to be emptied by a professional.

Long or short, fluffy or hairless, the cat's tail should also be examined for bumps and sores remembering that the base of the tail often harbors parasites and that the tail or nub does have nerve endings and a blood supply, so it can sustain injuries.

Throughout your assessment, check the cat's **skin and coat** for flaking or excessive shedding. The right brush can feel like a massage and help stimulate oil glands as well as prevent fur balls. If you notice anything that is irregular or abnormal for your cat, seek a professional veterinary opinion, and sometimes even a second opinion!

See Section III for Head-to-Tail Worksheet to keep you on track with home exams.

Also see page 208 in the pet safety section for a handy chart.

Basic Signs of Illness or Injury

During a head-to-tail check-up – or at any time – if you notice the following signs, the cat's health needs to be addressed. Don't be concerned about memorizing a list of symptoms. Think about when you yourself have not felt your best...what did you experience? It may not be that different from your cat except she won't tell you – rather she'll probably hide! It therefore is your task to seek out anything that is not right with your pet through weekly head-to-tail exams.

In the pages that follow, you will learn how to deal with these situations. The information below is your check list for determining the basic signs of illness or injury in a cat:

- Redness
- Swelling
- Tenderness/Lameness
- Open sores
- Bleeding, pus or discharge from any orifice or wound
- Breathing difficulties
- Rapid or decreased heart rate
- Excessive panting and squinting (which can be a sign of pain in cats)
- Slow CRT
- Abnormal temperature or hydration level
- Frequent or infrequent urination
- Any kind of unproductive straining to urinate or defecate
- Vomiting/diarrhea/constipation
- Restlessness
- Inability to walk
- Distended abdomen
- Lethargy
- Change in eating habits
- Anything that is not normal for YOUR cat may be ABNORMAL

Signs requiring Immediate Veterinary Care

Not All-inclusive but if you notice any of the following, seek immediate veterinary help:

- Severe bleeding or bleeding that doesn't stop in 5 minutes.
- Coughing up blood or bleeding from nose, eyes, ears, mouth or rectum
- Inability to urinate or defecate
- 1st time seizure or unusually long seizure
- Heatstroke
- Difficulty breathing
- Eye injuries
- Fractured bones
- Vomit / diarrhea with blood or recurrence (more than twice in 24 hours)
- Obvious pain or poisoning
- Staggering
- Refuse to drink for more than 24 hours

Remember that communication with your Veterinarian is always important and you should always feel comfortable seeking out their guidance, expertise and assistance.

Think Safety Before You Rush to the Rescue

You are no help to an injured animal if you get bitten or injured yourself. Take a breath and think. Kind of like you learned so many years ago, "Look both ways before you cross the street!" Prior to performing many pet first-aid techniques, it may be necessary to muzzle your cat or wrap her in a towel in order for you to safely offer assistance. Even the sweetest of animals may nip when he is scared or in pain. Practice safety first and remember that animals are very perceptive, picking up on your emotions. If you do not feel confident enough to help, you are better off getting the animal quickly to someone who can.

Restraining & Muzzling Techniques

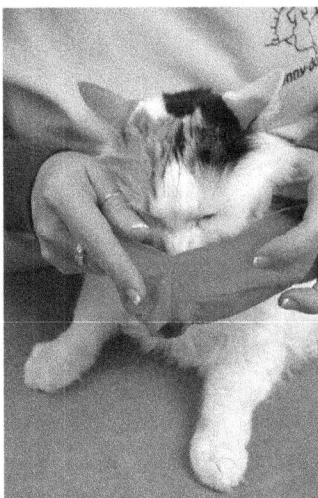

Rule number one is that you - the handler - must be in control. Make sure you have the cat in an enclosed area so that you are not struggling with her attempts to get away while you are trying to treat an injury. In other words, make sure doors, windows, gates, etc. are closed and there is no chance for escape.

Cats, when injured, tend to fight or flee, so coax them into a bathroom and shut the door. If your cat crawls under the sofa or bed while choking and then goes unconscious, you'll have to move the furniture before you can get to your pet – which wastes precious time. Cats settle best, (but no guarantees so practicing ahead helps), when you wrap them in a towel because it helps them feel more secure, but they may need to be muzzled to prevent them from biting you.

Photo by Sunny-dog Ink

Generally the best form of restraint is the least amount needed. For cats that might be scruffing -- grasping the loose skin at the nape of your cat's neck with a firm hold while resting your forearm again their back (see page 31 under Proper Handling & Restraint). Make sure your hand is close to the head and ears. If you hold the scruff too far down (towards the shoulders), kitty can turn her head and bite. With your other hand, hold the back legs stretching them backwards to restrain the cat. A commercially-made muzzle works best for cats.

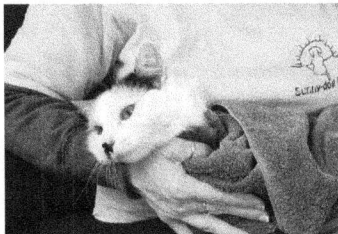

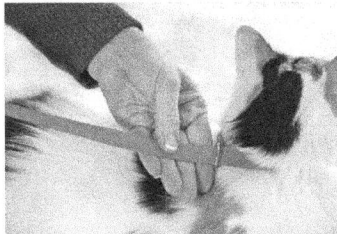

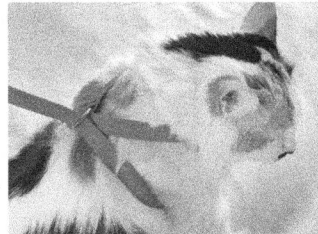

Photos by Sunny-dog Ink

Never leave a muzzled cat unattended -- she is defenseless. If a muzzled animal experiences breathing difficulty, vomiting or seizures, they could easily suffocate. Remove muzzle immediately if such signs or symptoms occur.

Additionally, restraint can include getting kitty gently and safely into her crate or carrier so that she can be transported for help.

How to Transport & Carry an Injured Cat

If kitty is too injured to be placed inside a carrier, remove the top (if possible) or place the animal into a sturdy cardboard box with an open top. Although no one likes to think of kitty on a cookie sheet, small boards like cookie sheets, pull-out counter cutting boards and the lids from plastic storage boxes all make excellent boards to secure a cat. Just secure her at the hips and shoulders by tying with a triangular bandage or even gauze out of your cat's first-aid kit. *Do not attempt to carry a cat on any kind of improvised backboard device if she is struggling or resisting the restraint as this could cause additional injury.*

Assembling a Cat First-Aid Kit

Just like a plumber or a carpenter, every task becomes easier if you have the right tool for the job, so aside from possessing life-saving skills, it is vital to have your pet's tool kit -- a Cat First-Aid Kit -- at your fingertips…at home, in the car and in your disaster preparedness supply.

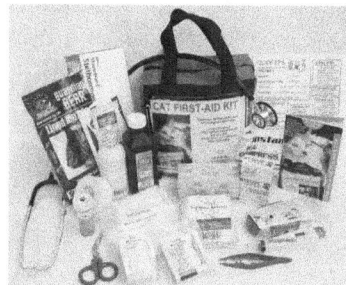

Photo by Sunny-dog Ink

All cat first-aid kits should include:

- 2" X 2" gauze squares to control bleeding
- Rolled gauze (2-3" varying sizes) to secure gauze squares in place, bandage a wound or make a temporary muzzle
- Adhesive tape or self-adhering bandage – to secure rolled gauze in place
- Styptic powder and cotton swabs to control minor bleeding
- Bandage scissors or blunt-nose scissors to carefully remove bandages, cut proper lengths of bandaging materials or safely trim pet fur
- Tweezers - to pull ticks or remove debris from a wound
- Hydrogen peroxide (3%) to clean a wound site
- Eye wash or sterile saline solution to flush minor wounds and clean eyes
- Chlorhexidine (commonly found as Hibiclens®) to flush cuts and wounds
- Cold pack to aid in heat stroke, swollen joints, burns and bee stings (apply to site of injury but frequently remove to prevent over-chilling/frostbite to the area)
- Antibiotic ointment or Vitamin E gel or pure aloe vera gel to soothe and promote healing. Apply externally to minor cuts, scrapes and insect bites (not animal bites). If using medicated ointments, use the least amount necessary making sure it soaks in so that your pet does not ingest when licking because he will.
- Dose syringe (needle-less syringe) or eye dropper to administer medications and other liquids

- Digital thermometer & lubricant to check your cat's temperature
- Antihistamine tablets (Diphenhydramine or Benadryl® - not containing cetirizine, acetaminophen or pseudoephedrine) for bee stings or allergic reactions (if you can find gel capsules, also have a straight pin in your kit to prick them open. You can then squeeze the liquid under your pet's tongue. Anything that is absorbed sublingually gets into the system even faster than swallowed.)
- Electrolyte solution to aid in re-hydration. Pedialyte®-type products are fine as long as they do not contain xylitol, an artificial sweetener harmful to pets. Sports-type drinks contain too much sugar and are not recommended. Pedialyte® should be diluted with water 50/50. Having salt & honey to make your own is also a smart idea (see recipe on page 151).
- Nylon slip-leash to devise a figure 8-harness.
- Towel or blanket can be used to cover a pet to maintain body heat and/or elevate his hindquarters to promote circulation. Can also be used to wrap the kitty for restraint purposes.
- Honey or Karo® Syrup
- This Cat First-Aid Handbook to assist with the important details you need to know.
- Important names and phone numbers including your Veterinarian, nearest veterinary emergency center, animal poison control, helpful neighbors, police and fire departments.

HOW TO GIVE YOUR CAT AN INJECTION OR SUB-Q FLUIDS

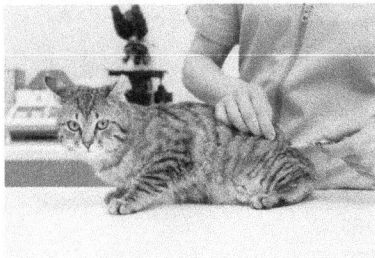

These techniques are best learned from your Veterinarian, but as a reminder once you've been properly instructed...

1) Draw the precise dose of medication into the syringe by placing the hub of proper sized needle into the vial's rubber stopper. Vial should be held upside down to a 45° angle for best effect.

2) Point the needle towards the ceiling and tap the syringe with your finger making sure any and all bubbles move to the top of syringe near the needle.

3) Slightly press the plunger on the syringe to force out any air. When you notice a teeny tiny drop of medication come out the tip of the needle, the air is out and you are set to inject.

4) Get yourself and your pet in a comfortable position and project calmness. Animals are very perceptive and will pick up on any stress you have. Gently pull up on the loose skin at the nape of your cat's neck or shoulders with one hand, while inserting the needle horizontally with the other. Take care to note your finger location and be careful to not insert the needle all the way through the cat's skin and into your own finger.

5) Smoothly press on plunger and release full complement of medication under your cat's skin, then remove needle.

6) Depending on the medication, your Veterinarian might advise you to rub the area afterwards to soothe the sting and help deliver the meds into your cat's body.

7) Properly dispose of needle in a "Sharps" container and give your kitty cat a little extra TLC for being such a good patient!

ALWAYS use the proper gauge (size) needle and amount of medication as dosed by your Veterinarian and report any usual reactions to him immediately. FYI...the smaller the number, the thicker the needle!

For sub-cutaneous fluid injections, which are usually due to severe dehydration or chronic kidney disease, the technique is very similar to giving an injection of insulin or other medication, but is done in larger quantities. Due to the amount given, it may take several hours for the fluid to be absorbed, so always check at the injection site and at the belly to make sure fluids have been fully absorbed before giving another dose. The reason you also need to check at the belly is gravity which can cause the fluid to accumulate at the under carriage.

Again, this technique is best learned from your veterinary professional and may vary slightly from pet to pet, but as a reminder:

1) Place hub proper needle with plastic cover still in place over the tip of the syringe. Some brands have threads and actually screw together.

2) Fluids generally come in plastic bags or glass bottles. You may be instructed to draw fluids from the same container several times and/or for several days. Never re-draw fluids from a container that you have used to inject fluids into your dog or cat or you will contaminate the fluid! Always use a sterile needle. Using an 18 gauge pink needle to draw fluids and a 20 gauge yellow needle to inject into your cat will minimize confusion, but go on the advice of your Veterinarian.

3) Clean the rubber stopper or port of the bag with chlorhexidine or betadine. Alcohol takes 30 minutes of contact to kill bacteria, so it's not the best choice.

4) Lay bag of fluid on a flat surface, remove plastic cover from needle and insert needle into rubber stopper horizontally so as not to puncture neck of fluid bag. Never use fluid if it appears cloudy through the bag.

5) Draw into syringe the appropriate amount of fluid. Remove needle from stopper, place plastic cover back over needle and remove needle from the barrel of the syringe to replace with sterile needle needed to give the injection.

6) When ready to inject, push plunger to release any air and gently grab fold of skin along pet's back or neck with your left hand if you are right handed (southpaws reverse). Inject needle into skin making sure blood does not appear. If it does, you have hit a blood vessel, so back out needle and try again.

7) Once needle is in place, release the fold of skin and push on plunger to inject fluid. It is often helpful to steady the barrel of the syringe with one hand while you press plunger with the other.

8) Safely dispose of needles, properly store any unused fluids and as always... give your four-legged patient a special belly rub or ear scratch for being a good patient.

How to use a Stethoscope

Find a quiet space for you and your pet, then...
1) Angle the binaurals (ear pieces) forward so as to be at the same angle as your ear canal.

2) Moisten the pet's hair with water or rubbing alcohol to reduce the sound of hair rustling against the heads.

3) Have pet sit or stand. Lying on their side may cause the heart to rub against the chest wall. Place the bell (larger round disc) on the left side of the dog where his elbow touches his chest if it were gently pulled back. Cat hearts are smaller and vibrate at a higher frequency, so the heart is better heard using the diaphragm (smaller side of round disc) and placing it directly on the cat's sternum (center of chest).

Average Heart & Respiration Rate For Cats	
Species	**Average Heart & Respiration Rate**
Cats	*160 - 200 Heart Beats Per Minute* *20 - 40 Breaths Per Minute*
Please Note: *Very large cats and geriatric animals may have slower respirations. Rule of thumb is that the bigger and older the cat, the slower their pulse or respiraton. The smaller and younger the cat, the faster their breathing and pulse rate.*	

HEART BEAT If you do not hear anything, administer CPR and get to your Veterinarian or Animal ER immediately! Swishing or a vibration could indicate a murmur, so please have pet seen by a medical professional.

RESPIRATORY SOUNDS Anything other than rhythmic breaths requires diagnosis by your Veterinarian, including wheezing, gurgling or whistling sounds. Don't delay.

Don't Just Stand There! How to Handle a Choking Cat

CHOKING

CONDITION OVERVIEW:
When an object gets lodged in front of the trachea (windpipe) instead of passing down the esophagus, it can prevent air from getting to the pet's lungs and can cause them to go unconscious – a life-threatening condition.

Cats are more apt to choke on a furball or a piece of ribbon, yarn, dental floss or thread. Do not yank such an object out of your cat's mouth. Occasionally a sewing needle may be attached to the other end! Even if you don't fear a sharp object could be attached to the string, there are small nodules in the body as well as the intestines which can become entangled. If you can't safely retrieve the long object from kitty's mouth, cut it off so she cannot swallow more, and get her to the Veterinarian right away.

PREVENTIVE MEASURES INCLUDE:
Get down on all fours and look at your house and yard from your cat's perspective. Anything in paw's reach could end up inside your cat:

Common Household Items that can be swallowed:
- Push pins, staples, buttons, rubber bands, toothpicks
- Dental floss, hair ties & ribbons

SIGNS & SYMPTOMS:
- Loud noise or cough as an animal exhales
- Rasping noise as he inhales
- Gagging or retching as if trying to vomit
- Pawing at the mouth
- Drooling
- Outward stretching of the neck
- Staggering and eventually rapid/shallow breathing
- Pale/blue gums
- Collapse

NOTE: If the cat's tongue is swollen it may have resulted in choking due to a blocked airway; but the choking may have also been induced by an allergic reaction.

WHAT YOU MAY NEED:
You must remain calm and act quickly.

Possibly tweezers, or forceps to reach into a tiny feline mouth and grab an object but see what you are grabbing! Be aware however that your kitty Heimlich-like skills most often help you come to the rescue!

WHAT TO DO:

Initially, give the cat a few moments to cough. She may expel the object on her own. If the cause of choking is not alleviated by the cat's own coughing action, a careful sweep of the mouth with your fingers to dislodge the object is recommended if the animal will let you safely do so. Make sure you can see inside the animal's mouth before you attempt to move anything. Do not reach without looking as you could push the object deeper, tear laryngeal tissue by pulling an embedded object or even get bitten.

With your hand coming from behind and overhead, place thumb and index finger in cheek where upper and lower jaw meet to open kitty's mouth.

If the obstruction can't be safely removed, try one of the techniques below:

Abdominal Compression (Kitty Heimlich-like Maneuver)
Standing behind and over your kitty, place the flats of two fingers in the soft part of the stomach just behind the last rib. You should be able to feel a triangular area on his abdomen that would be the rib cage. Brace the cat's back with your opposite hand and compress your fingers towards you hand with 5 quick thrusts... and compress the abdomen with 5 quick thrusts similar to the Heimlich Technique performed on humans.

Chest Thrusts
An alternative method is to place several fingers on each side of the cat's chest and thrust inward, pushing in the direction you want the object to go – out the mouth. After 2-3 thrusts, give the kitty a moment to cough and/or look in her mouth to see if the object is now reachable. If not, repeat.

You may also try the Heimlich-like Manuever for cats using just the flats of two fingers (instead of your fist) in the soft part of the belly and bracing the pet with your other hand on his back, pulling up towards that hand.

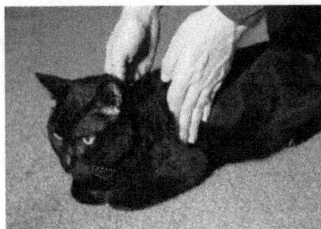

Photo by: Sunny-dog Ink

Unconscious Choking Victim
Place cat on her side with the flat pads of several fingers over her heart and compress to squeeze the lungs. By squeezing air out of the lungs, the goal is to create a force that will move the object into the mouth so that you can then reach it. Alternate these thrusts with rescue breathing & CPR if it takes more than 2 minutes to accomplish (brain cells start to die within 3 minutes without oxygen) so get immediate veterinary help. Details are described in the next section for rescue breathing and CPR.

RESCUE BREATHING & CPCR

	COMPRESSION: BREATH RATIO	NORMAL PULSE
NEONATES (Newborns)	1:1 Compress Chest 1/2" - 1"	120 - 200 bpm
SMALL (Under 20 lbs.)	30:2 Compress Chest 1/2" - 1"	120 - 200 bpm

CONDITION OVERVIEW:

Cardio Pulmonary Resuscitation (CPR) is the most commonly known method of artificial life support. Recent research has led to the advancement of a faster more efficient method referred to as Cardio Pulmonary Cerebral Resuscitation (CPCR). Both of these techniques utilize a combination of chest compressions and artificial respirations, however CPCR focuses more on chest compressions and less on artificial respirations. CPCR utilizes the theory that the action of compressing the chest facilitates the movement of oxygen (that is already in the cat's body) through the lungs, lessening the number of times you will need to give breaths via the nasal passage. Oxygen moves through the body via the blood, so if you are promoting circulation, you are also moving oxygen via the bloodstream throughout the unconscious animal's body. Classic CPR uses a combination of five to fifteen compressions (depending on the size of the animal) and the administration of two breaths, whereas the more efficient CPCR procedure calls for 30 vigorous chest compressions for every 2 breaths given.

PREVENTIVE MEASURES/CAUSES INCLUDE:

- Smoke Inhalation
- Heat Stroke or hyperthermia (internal body temperature of 104° F or higher)
- Electrocution
- Hit by Car
- Drowning
- Poisoning
- Choking
- Gunshot
- Hypoglycemia (low blood sugar)

SIGNS & SYMPTOMS:

Cat has lost consciousness and both heartbeat and breathing have stopped.

Know that even under the best circumstances (in an animal ER with trained and experienced staff, medications, access to oxygen, tracheal tubes and IV catheters) the outcome may not always be successful, but how can you not try if an animal is depending on you? According to the American Heart Association, human survival rates range from 6.4% - 20%. In a hospital setting, on average 10% cats are successfully resuscitated via CPCR.

Although you may have taken a human CPR course, cats don't share our anatomy. The concept is the same, but the technique is different. You may be familiar with the "ABC's of CPR" (airway, breathing, circulation); recent studies by the American Heart Association have shown that keeping the blood flowing to the brain (circulation) is more valuable as a life-saving tool than the administration of artificial respiration. In light of this research, the newest recommended protocol is "CAB" (circulation, airway, breathing) placing the emphasis on compressions over breaths . Following this recommendation from the American Heart Association, the veterinary community has also adopted this new protocol.

NOTE: Cats rarely go into cardiac arrest with "shockable" rhythms. Even if you have access to a defibrillator, it is NOT advised!

CAB = CIRCULATION, AIRWAY, BREATHING

WHAT YOU MAY NEED:
A hard surface on which to perform chest compressions (ground, table, floor, board underneath cat in a back seat for instance).

Calm, cool, you and the means to lift and transport the cat to the Animal ER.

Another person if available and willing to assist. Helping hands can be useful even if they are not trained in first aid or don't possess animal experience. As long as the person is calm, he or she can assist you in getting materials, lifting the kitty or even driving to the Animal ER while you tend to your pet!

WHAT TO DO:

- Place cat on a flat surface on his side and slightly extend her head by pulling back on the chin to stretch out her throat/tracheal area. Not only does this straighten out the airway but also minimizes your chance of blowing air into her stomach rather than lungs.

- Take the cat's front leg, gently bending it at the elbow and bring it towards the chest. This is a gentle movement bending the animal's elbow at the joint. Where the elbow touches the chest is the proper spot to place your hands for compressions.

- Compress approximately 1/3 the width of the chest diameter. You should feel ribs, then press a lung before you compress the heart to effectively create circulation.

- When giving breaths, use 1-2 hands to seal off mouth and breathe directly into the cat's nostrils. For neonates, use a small puff breath only. Remember... if you need to perform CPCR, the pet is theoretically "dead," so although we don't want to break a rib, the important thing is to get that life-giving blood & oxygen circulating. Properly performed, ribs break only 1.6% of the time which should give you some relief.

Never perform CPCR or rescue breathing on a conscious animal!

CPCR Technique

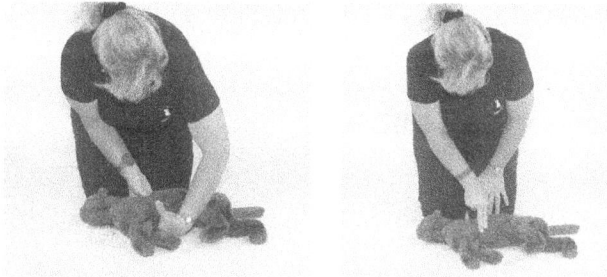

Photos by: Sunny-dog Ink

For Cats

Follow above CPCR technique but place their chest in the palm of your hand (use two hands if the animal's chest is too wide). Four fingers should be on one side, your thumb on the other side of the chest so that compressions will gently but directly impact the heart. Squeeze your fingers together to compress the chest. Follow with 2 breaths and repeat. Cats do not require as much pressure during chest compressions but tune in and visualize to make sure you are applying just enough pressure to squeeze blood out of the heart then releasing to allow circulation and refilling of the heart before you squeeze again. You need to be the pump that the animal's heart cannot be at this time.

For neonates (kittens -- hours or days old):

Follow the same CPCR technique, but administer one compression and one puff breath at a time. If your hand covers the entire torso (when trying to attempt chest compressions as mentioned above), place your thumb on one-side of the chest and use only two fingers (index finger and middle finger) on the other side. Squeeze the chest with the flat tips of your fingers.

NOTE: Rapid initiation of CPCR is critical and must be started within 4 minutes after the heart stops beating to avoid brain damage.

Quickly transport feline patient to the nearest animal emergency center or veterinary hospital. Realize that you may not get the cat to breathe or resume a heart beat on her own and may need to continue CPCR while someone else drives. Do not stop administering CPCR until the cat shows signs of recovery or until a veterinary professional can take over.

If you are able to continue compressions on the way to the hospital, a firm floor like in an SUV or Station Wagon is best to lay the pet on. If you are doing compressions on a cushioned back seat, find a board or something sturdy to place between the cat and the cushion to aid squeezing the heart. Otherwise you'll just be pushing the injured animal into the seat cushion. If you cannot locate a board quickly, place your other hand/fist underneath the pet to press against.

RESCUE BREATHING (aka Mouth-to-Snout Resuscitation)

CONDITION OVERVIEW:
Cat is not breathing. Lungs have filled with fluid, can't receive oxygen due to a blockage, swelling or other injury/illness. Cat is in a life-threatening situation!

PREVENTIVE MEASURES/CAUSES INCLUDE:
- Allergic Reactions (such as bee stings)
- Choking
- Collapsed or Punctured Lung
- Drowning
- Pneumonia
- Poisoning
- Smoke Inhalation
- Trauma

SIGNS & SYMPTOMS:
Cat is not breathing – no detected "rise & fall" to the chest.

WHAT YOU MAY NEED:
A calm demeanor (animals are perceptive and pick up on our emotions, even when unconscious).

Another person if available and willing to assist. Helping hands can be useful even if they are not trained in first aid or don't possess animal experience. As long as the person is calm, he or she can assist you in getting materials, lifting an animal or even driving to the Animal hospital while you tend to your pet!

Means to lift and transport pet to Animal ER.

WHAT TO DO:
- Rescue breathing in cats is done via the nasal passage (not the mouth as in humans). Their "smile line" goes farther around the face making it difficult to seal off the mouth and administer breaths without losing air through the sides of the mouth.
- Always make sure the mouth is adequately closed and sealed.
- Evaluate the size of the kitty to judge the volume of artificial breaths to be administered. CPCR is not an exact science, so tune in to your cat and stay focused. It is important that the lungs are not over-inflated. It is best to pay attention to your cat ahead of time noticing how much her chest rises as she sleeps or rests to give you a frame of reference.

Rescue Breathing Technique

With the catt on his side, gently close her mouth with one or two of your hands until her "smile line" – the portion of her lips that wrap around her face – are sealed.

- For a cat, you may just be using your thumb and index finger to make this seal.

- Make a tight seal with your mouth around the nose and deliver breaths.

Sealing a cat's mouth in preparation for Rescue Breathing

Deliver two slow full breaths into the nostrils, making sure you ventilate (actually see the lungs rise but just the slightest movement is sufficient) the animal and allow time for exhalation (lungs to fall into relaxed position) between the breaths.

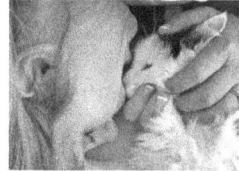

Photo by: Sunny-dog Ink

Basic Cat First-Aid Techniques: Injuries & Illnesses

Now that you have a good understanding of vital signs, breathing, circulation and choking management, we will discuss the basic first-aid techniques for an assortment of other injuries and illnesses that could happen to an animal in your care.

Important…First-aid is not intended to replace professional veterinary care. The administration of first-aid is done in order to prevent further injury to the animal in your care and to alleviate pain and distress. Follow-up and continued treatment by a competent veterinary professional is imperative in most cases.

Familiarize yourself with this section for ease of use when you need it.

Like both the Choking & Rescue Breathing/CPCR portions of this book, each Injury or Illness has 5 sub-categories:

1) CONDITION OVERVIEW (explains the illness or injury).

2) PRECAUTIONS/CAUSES (how you may prevent and/or what might cause the specific injury or illness to help you assess if it is in fact what your cat may be experiencing).

3) SIGNS & SYMPTOMS (how your cat may be reacting if he does have this condition - he does not have to exhibit all the signs to be in distress).

4) WHAT YOU NEED (tools needed from your cat first-aid kit).

5) WHAT TO DO (action you should take, often including a trip to your Veterinarian) to help you help your cat recover.

To assist in preventing the worst from happening, you will find more detailed precautions to take in the SAFETY Section in the front of this book. It is the authors' hopes that if you stay aware to what might cause injury and illness that you will be better prepared to help your dog or cat avoid catastrophe.

A NOTE ABOUT HOMEOPATHY... Along with more traditional first-aid tips, homeopathic suggestions are offered in the Injuries & Illness section of this book. As with any other offering, your Veterinarian who has the luxury of physically seeing and knowing your pet is your best source for advice but listed are methods that may make your dog or cat feel more comfortable prior to seeking veterinary care or with your professional's approval, along with other treatment.

Homeopathic remedies include tinctures, small pellets, pills and mists. Homeopathy works on the premise that "like cures like." For example, an approach to dealing with bee stings, rashes and other swellings would be administering *Apis Meliffica* which comes from the female honey bee (the females by the way are the only ones with venom). Homeopathy embraces the notion that the body can heal itself and that symptoms are a sign that the body is in a state of repair attempting to restore its own health. By giving a very small and diluted amount of a similar substance (herb, essence) the body's natural defenses are triggered to heal itself.

Homeopathics can often be administered along with other traditional treatments, and typically 30c of a homeopathic remedy is the highest dosage obtainable without a prescription. One "c" is equal to one part of the original diluted 99 times, so 30c is one part diluted 99 X 30.

Other identifying doses you may see include:

X = 1 : 9 dilution

C = 1 : 99 dilution

LM = 1 : 10,000 dilution

Best absorbed when placed under the tongue or on the gums, homeopathic remedies may be found as tinctures but also on sugar pills where just a drop of the remedy has been placed. It is preferable to avoid touching the pill by crushing it between two spoons and placing under your pet's tongue, or... to dissolve the pill in a drop of distilled water and then suck into a syringe to again be delivered under the tongue for best effects.

Once a good response is achieved with homeopathics, you do not continue with higher doses but back off frequency and amount.

Please Note:

If you feel uncomfortable performing any steps suggested in this book on an animal needing care, instead...get the pet to immediate veterinary help. Cats are very perceptive and react to our body language and stress, so if you are fearful, it will be better for both you and the animal if you stay calm and obtain immediate assistance.

What you are reading in the following pages are suggested guidelines suitable for most pets under normal circumstances. Your Veterinarian, Nutritionist, Behaviorist, Homeopathic or Alternative Medicine Specialist's recommendations should be taken over those presented in this book as that individual has the advantage of seeing your pet personally and knowing their unique history.

Injuries & Illnesses:

ABSCESSES

CONDITION OVERVIEW:
Abscesses develop when germs get caught beneath the skin as in the case of puncture wounds.

PREVENTIVE MEASURES/CAUSES:
- Animal bites/fights with other cats!
- Nails, tacks, staples, splinters
- Gunshot

SIGNS & SYMPTOMS:
- Possible limp depending on location
- Hot, red, swollen area
- Open wound with pus
- Elevated Body Temperature

WHAT YOU MAY NEED:
- Thermometer
- Blunt nosed scissors
- Chlorhexidine, Betadine® or anti-bacterial soap
- Epsom Salt
- Gauze Squares
- Warm Water
- Warm Compress
- E-Collar to prevent licking

WHAT TO DO:
Carefully clip fur from area surrounding wound with blunt-nosed scissors, and wash away any discharge with a Chlorhexidine-type product. Soak a washcloth or gauze in Epsom Salt Solution (1/4 cup Epsom Salt to 1 quart very warm water), squeeze out slightly and place on top of the swollen tissue for 5 minutes three to five times a day. Wash as needed. Abscesses often become quite painful and need to be drained by a professional who can also prescribe antibiotics to heal completely, so see your Veterinarian. A blood test could also be necessary to determine if the infection has entered the blood stream.

NOTE: Never place a hot compress in the pits or groin area as you will overheat the animal -- these are locations to major arteries (Femoral/Brachial). If you can't avoid major arteries due to location of the abscess, seek professional medical help for your cat at once.

ALLERGIES

CONDITION OVERVIEW:
Cats can be allergic to many of the same things we are: dust mites, fleas, pollen, grasses and food. Often though instead of coughing or sneezing, cats SCRATCH. They may also lick their paws or chew on their tails. An allergy is a hypersensitivity to something your cat comes in contact with. It is the way their immune system responds to what is irritating them.

PREVENTIVE MEASURES/CAUSES:
- Anything on the floor or ground can soak into your cat's paws or be consumed when she grooms. Using cat-friendly cleaners, insecticides and other products can help eliminate irritants.

- Avoid cat foods containing wheat, corn and soy as well as table scraps.

- Pollens, aerosol air fresheners and anything with a scent can irritate.

SIGNS & SYMPTOMS:
- Scratching or licking
- Red irritated skin
- Hair loss in patches
- Sneezing, Coughing, Discharge from eyes or nose
- Change in skin or coat – flaky skin, dull fur; body odor

WHAT YOU MAY NEED:
- Oatmeal Shampoo
- Pure Aloe Vera Gel
- Diphenhydramine/Benedryl® (not containing Cetirizine, Acetaphetamine or Pseudoephedrine)
- Possible change in diet
- Non-allergenic laundry detergent
- Scissors
- E-Collar or sock and bandaging material

WHAT TO DO:
A Veterinary visit and subsequent testing may be the only way to determine the root of the allergy and best course of action to take. If an irritation exists, you may try eliminating wheat and/or corn from your cat's diet (removing only one ingredient at a time for several weeks to determine which, if either, is responsible for the allergy), switch to a novel (unfamiliar) protein such as lamb or venison, and give Fluffy a soothing oatmeal or aloe bath.

Alleviate symptoms with Diphenhydramine (Benadryl®) – 1mg per pound of cat's body weight, but always check with your Veterinarian first to make sure it won't interact with any other conditions your pet has or medications she takes. Never use time-released capsules for pets. If using liquid Benedryl®, 5 ml should equal 12.5 mg of diphenydramine, so...dosage = .4ml / lbs. pet weight

For sore patches of skin, trim fur close to the skin with blunt-nosed scissors. Unless you are a groomer or Veterinarian, it may be difficult to use a razor on a moving animal without causing further harm. Clean the area with anti-bacterial soap, pat dry and apply aloe vera gel or hydrocortisone cream. Then prevent pet from licking or chewing, possibly by wearing the awfully named "cone of shame" (E- or cone collar. Do look around. There are many more comfortable versions available.). You might also try placing a human sock over the wound to prevent licking or apply a bandage with the overwrap containing a cat-safe anti-lick product.

ANAL GLANDS / ANAL SAC PROBLEMS

CONDITION OVERVIEW:
Has Tiger been doing the butt-scoot boogie lately or dashing around the house pausing only to lick his backside? Anal sacs are scent glands that normally release small amounts of fluid through tiny openings when your pet defecates. They contain a strong-smelling fluid that pets use to "mark" their territory and identify each other. From this information, they can tell each other's sex, interest in mating and what they had for lunch! When, for unknown reasons, they become impacted, infected or create an abscess, your cat scoots or licks to alleviate the discomfort.

PREVENTIVE MEASURES/CAUSES:
- Human food can cause stools to be unusually soft making fluid more likely to build up so avoid table scraps and make sure pets get fiber.
- Doing a weekly head-to-tail check-up and paying attention to your cat's habits could alert you during the early stages before this condition, with unknown causes, becomes a bigger problem.
- Add 1/2 teaspoon daily of pumpkin puree or shredded raw carrot to your pet's diet. When the fiber is eliminated through bathroom habits, glands often express themselves.

SIGNS & SYMPTOMS:
- Chewing or licking obsessively under the tail
- Butt scooting
- Red or swollen anus

WHAT YOU MAY NEED:
- Rubber or Latex-free gloves
- Soft cloth or gauze square
- Shampoo or antibacterial soap for clean-up
- Pumpkin Puree or change of diet

WHAT TO DO:
Feed pumpkin puree (not pumpkin pie mix with added sugar and spices) -- 1 Tablespoon for a cat. Do not over feed the pumpkin as it is also a cure for constipation. Another option might be adding probiotics to your cat's diet. You should see improvements in about four weeks.

A temporary and much-needed fix however, is to express the glands.

Your Veterinarian or groomer should be adept at emptying these pesky sacs on your cat, but if you feel confident enough to try, follow these steps:

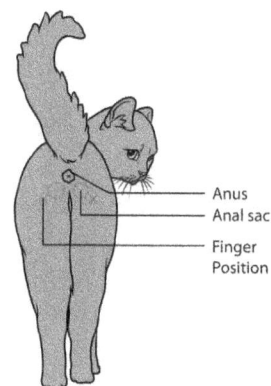
Anus
Anal sac
Finger Position

- Take your pet to the tub or a place that is easy to clean (Yep, this is a messy task).
- With rubber or latex gloves on your hands, kneel or stand at your cat's side, lift his tail with one hand and hold a cloth in the other hand to catch the secretions.
- For cats…they extend to four and eight o'clock. If the sacs are full, you will feel two hard bulges, not much larger than a pea. With the hand that is holding the cloth, place your thumb and forefinger on either side of the anal opening at the positions mentioned above, and gently press inward and upward in a semi-circular motion as if tracing a clock dial.. Just make sure the anus is covered with the cloth. The fluid may be thin or thick and varies from yellow to light gray or brown.
- If nothing comes out, adjust your finger positions, but if you still come up dry, consult your Veterinarian. Pushing too hard may be painful to your pet.

ARTHRITIS

CONDITION OVERVIEW:

Degenerative joint disease or Osteoarthritis usually occurs after years of wear and tear on the joints but can affect a pet at any age. Large dogs are most vulnerable but kitties too can feel the pain. It can affect one or more joints and is found in one out of five dogs at some point during their lifetime. Once your cat gets arthritis, she will definitely require veterinary care to alleviate pain.

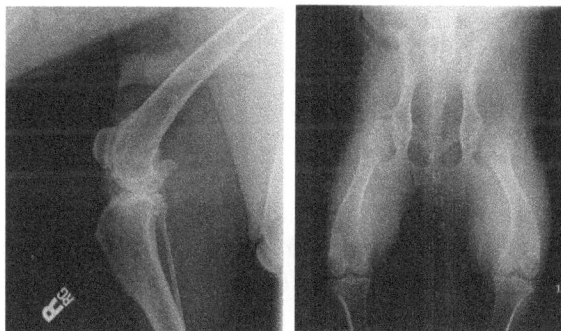
Photos Courtesy of Sunny-dog Ink

PREVENTIVE MEASURES/CAUSES:
- Obesity
- Genetics
- Hip Dysplasia, Cruciate Ligament injuries, Patella Luxation can contribute

SIGNS & SYMPTOMS:
- Laying around more
- Pain or difficulty getting up; flopping when laying down
- Moaning with movement
- Labored, stiff movements

In some cases, constipation could be a symptom of arthritis! Since it may hurt kitty to get into the appropriate #2 squat position, she may not go and this may back her system up. The result is constipation but the cause could be the pain of arthritis.

WHAT YOU MAY NEED:
- Veterinary assessment to determine course of action (medication, therapy, light exercise, massage)
- Supportive pet bed (egg crate foam or firm mattress) in a draft free location. Too soft beds and nesting cushions are difficult to get up and out of.
- Non-slippery floor surfaces or toe/paw grips for traction.

WHAT TO DO:
Keeping your cat at a healthy weight along with providing her regular gentle exercise (following a feather toy, playing with another cat) to keep the joints fluid and the muscles strong is your best course of action.

Make sure your cat's bed is made of material she doesn't sink into too deeply making it difficult to get up and out of, and make sure it is placed in a draft-free location.

Provide ramps to make stair climbing easier. Placing a chair or low stool under a window will allow your feline friend to still enjoy her favorite sunny windowsill. An ottoman or bench seat by your bed will allow make it easier for her to snuggle with you. So many new products are on the market to help out pets, so do your research and find what works best for your house and your pet.

Consult your Veterinarian for medications that may take the edge off her pain. Follow your Veterinarian's instructions. New prescriptions often come to light, but always follow directions including any blood work or testing to catch any side effects early.

Glucosamine, Chondroitin, Methylsulfonylmethane (MSM) and Hyaluronic Acid are supplements that can help rebuild cartilage and joint fluids providing better movement for your cat. Speak with an expert about the possibilities or CBD and other option that may provide additional comfort as well.

BACK & DISC INJURIES

CONDITION OVERVIEW:
Cats vertebrae are like spools on a string that have elastic cushioning discs in between. Their limber spine allows them to perform graceful moves and also gives them their speed. The Dachshund's feline counterpart – the Munchkin – is therefore not as prone to disc injuries with her flexible feline physique.

PREVENTIVE MEASURES/CAUSES:
- Genetics
- Overweight cats more prone
- Provide ramps in place of stairs
- Falling, jumping, slipping or having an object fall on your pet
- Leaping on and off furniture

SIGNS & SYMPTOMS:
- Pain
- Inability to use hind legs or stand
- Walk with a wobbly gait or walk on the top of the paws instead of the pads due to loss of sensation

WHAT YOU MAY NEED:
- Board or surface you can carry cat on
- Triangular Bandage, strips of fabric or rope to secure kitty to board
- Honey or Karo® Syrup
- Gauze and bandaging supplies

WHAT TO DO:
Get the cat to veterinary help without causing further injury.

Check for breathing & pulse administering any first-aid or life-saving measures needed if injury was due to trauma (ie: stop bleeding, rub honey on the gums, treat for shock).

Slide flat board under the animal, keeping her as still as possible (Remember a calm soothing voice). Prevent movement as much as possible as struggling can damage the spinal cord. Secure the animal to the board with a triangular bandage or torn strips of cloth at the shoulders and hips. Place a towel over your cat's body and use fabric or gauze roll over the towel to the board or other surface to keep her secure. The last thing you want is for your cat to fall from the stretcher as you carry her.

Transport to a veterinary facility immediately.

NOTE: Please read section on how to transport an injured animal on page 99.

BALANCE (Loss of)

CONDITION OVERVIEW:
Known as Vestibular Syndrome, the symptoms can be upsetting to see when your precious feline is experiencing a loss of balance. It is often mistaken for poisoning, seizures or even a stroke and sometimes…there is never a definable cause. In medical speak, when Veterinarians can't determine the reason, the disease or syndrome is tagged idiopathic. Vestibular Syndrome can strike a cat at any age, but older ones are more prone.

What the Vestibular system does is helps the animal stay in equilibrium in relation to gravity. It conveys information to the muscles and controls eye movement so that images remain steady and in focus. This all takes place through mechanoreceptors found in the inner ear. Therefore, inner ear infections are a known cause for vestibular syndrome in cats and must be ruled out by your Veterinarian. Less common is a tumor on or near the Vestibular center of the brain stem.

PREVENTIVE MEASURES/CAUSES:
- Check your cat's ears weekly for signs of infection or debris and keep them clean.

SIGNS & SYMPTOMS:
- Head tilt, circling or falling all directed toward the same side
- Jerking of the eyes from side-to-side (aka Nystagmus)
- Vomiting
- Loss of appetite

WHAT YOU MAY NEED:
- Antacid prescribed by Veterinarian or 1 tsp Mylanta® for every 10-15 lbs pet weighs to curb nausea
- Needle-less syringe or eye dropper to administer antacid
- Due diligence to make sure your wobbly kitty doesn't fall or roam stray; secure windows, add gates to block off stairs and balconies and assess your home from your cat's point of view.

WHAT TO DO:
Get an immediate and thorough veterinary exam.

If the ear is found to be infected, treatment will be prescribed.

If the ear is free of infection, then you and your Veterinarian will determine if an MRI or CT Scan is advisable to rule out a tumor, or if the symptoms should be dealt with as if idiopathic in origin. Often the syndrome resolves on its own over the course of several weeks, and unfortunately there is no way to speed recovery. Anti-nausea and/or dizziness medications may be prescribed as well as fluids, especially if your furry patient cannot eat.

During this time you must keep your cat safe by making sure they can't fall down stairs, out open windows, off balconies or other such hazards, and never let your cat with vestibular syndrome roam freely outside.

BIRTHING PROBLEMS (Dystocia)

CONDITION OVERVIEW:
Although it is important to have your Vet help you through a pet's pregnancy, you probably won't need to hire a Lamaze Coach. Do remember though all those cats out there that never find permanent loving homes, and please spay and neuter your pets! The vast majority of births go smoothly, so resist the urge to step in unless you are really needed.

PREVENTIVE MEASURES/CAUSES:
- A planned C-section is preferable to an emergency one, so plan ahead and confer with your vet as to whether your cat might be at-risk.. Nothing is worse for the mom-to-be than to have to be rushed to the vet hospital in the middle of the night or to become exhausted because she has been unsuccessfully straining to deliver kittens, sometimes for hours. The kittens are more likely to survive if they haven't been stuck in the birth canal or had their placentas detached, so talk with your Veterinarian about the possibilities ahead of time.
- Litters consisting of just one kitten and litters containing an oversized kitten just might require a C-section and can be determined ahead of time through x-rays carefully obtained by your Veterinarian, so...remember to be a team player with your medical professional for the sake of your four-legged friend.

SIGNS & SYMPTOMS TO CALL THE VETERINARIAN RIGHT AWAY:
- Your cat passes a dark green fluid before delivery which means the kitty's lifeline (the placenta) may have become separated too soon.
- Your momma cat has been straining hard without delivering for more than an hour – the baby could be too large or in the wrong position to come out without assistance.
- Your female seems weak, nervous or restless for more than a half hour after the labor stops. There could still be another kitty waiting to see the world.
- Momma has muscle tremors days or weeks after giving birth, begins to vomit or has trouble standing up. These could be a sign of Eclampsia – a dangerous deficiency of calcium that sometimes occurs after giving birth.

WHAT YOU MAY NEED:
- Thermometer
- K-Y® or other water soluble jelly
- Disposable gloves
- Clean towels, lots of them and small ones like washcloths
- Blunt scissors or electric clippings for trimming fur
- Sharp Scissors for umbilical cord
- Iodine
- Rubbing alcohol
- Thread
- Bulb suction syringe
- Milk replacer, nursing bottles, eye dropper or needle-less syringe

SIGNS & SYMPTOMS THAT DELIVERY IS IMMINENT:
- Mammary gland enlargement and milk secretion (1 to 2 weeks prior to delivery)
- Restlessness, seeking seclusion, losing weight, nesting (12 to 24 hours prior to delivery)
- Rectal temp decreases to less than 99°F (8 to 24 hours prior to delivery)
- Straining & involuntary contractions of the abdominal muscles (Final stage as fetuses begin to move through the birth canal)

WHAT TO DO & WHEN YOU SHOULD OFFER ASSISTANCE:
If delivery hasn't occurred by 67th day, get to your Veterinarian.

If the neonate comes out only part-way despite the mom's efforts, grasp the emerging kitten with a clean washcloth and gently pull him free. Do not attempt to remove a neonate in this way if you cannot see both the front legs and head.

If mom doesn't instinctively tear off the amniotic sac within 30 seconds, carefully peel away the amniotic sac from around the neonate's face. Clean the mucus from kitten's mouth with your finger and then rub newborn vigorously with a clean cloth.

Encourage mom to lick her baby and sever the umbilical cord.

Mom doesn't bite the umbilical cord within one minute. This typically happens when the mother doesn't immediately remove the amniotic sac. To sever the umbilical cord, tie two pieces of embroidery thread (dipped in rubbing alcohol) around the umbilical cord. The first thread should be tied about 1 ½ inches from the tummy and the second should be tied about an inch farther down the umbilical cord from the first thread. Clean a pair of sharp bandage scissors with rubbing alcohol and snip the umbilical cord between the threads.

HOMEOPATHIC TIP:
If the pet is having difficulty with discharges, such as after a false pregnancy or following pyometra, *Pulsatilla* may be useful. Consult your Homeopathic Veterinarian in advance.

BLADDER CONTROL PROBLEMS

CONDITION OVERVIEW:
Incontinence occurs when your cat cannot voluntarily control the act of voiding their urine. Bladder control problems can be related to infections and kidney disease, so a trip to your pet's medical professional is the best place to start. Incontinent cats wet their beds, the floor where they nap, dribble urine and go in inappropriate places even when they know better. This is often seen in older pets and can be caused by an estrogen (females) or testosterone (males) deficiency since these hormones play a role in the muscle tone of the urethral sphincter. Additionally, males with prostate issues don't completely empty their bladders when they answer nature's call, so they are always partially full and feel the urge to go more frequently, and sometimes…just can't reach the appropriate location in time.

Urinating in the wrong place however, can sometimes but a behavioral issue due to a change or disruption in lifestyle. Did you recently change cat litter brands or have you not cleaned her box to kitty's satisfaction? Is a new pet now sharing the house, or has work been keeping you away longer hours? Does your kitty become timid when you raise your voice or overly excited when you arrive home? All of these situations can cause certain pets to go right then and there or seek out your new bedspread to take out their frustrations on. Ask your Veterinarian to refer you to an Animal Behaviorist if you are seeing a pattern and medical conditions have been ruled out.

PREVENTIVE MEASURES/CAUSES:
- Diabetes or Hypothyroidism
- Weakened muscle tone due to hormonal changes or age
- Prostate issues
- Urinary Tract Disease such as Feline Urological Syndrome
- Stones, crystals or debris accumulate in the bladder or urethra
- Tumors
- Spinal cord problems

SIGNS & SYMPTOMS:
- Urinating outside the litter box
- Damp or wet bedding or sleeping area
- Straining or crying when attempting to go
- Skin around genitals appears red/sore from the ammonia-like leaking; constant licking of the area
- Bloody or cloudy urine
- Increased thirst
- Increased frequency in visits to the litter box or asking to go outside (if an indoor/ outdoor kitty)

WHAT YOU MAY NEED:
- Veterinary visit for starters to diagnose problem.

WHAT TO DO:
Keep litter box clean and provide extra "bathrooms" for your cat upstairs and downstairs.

Take up water bowls two-hours before "lights out" and keep meals on a regular schedule.

Make any clean-up easier for you so that you won't become frustrated with your precious pet.

Line bedding with plastic and make sure everything is easily washable -- no dry clean only materials.

Kitty cat diapers can be worn but check them frequently so that irritating fluids don't scald your pet's skin.

BLEEDING INJURIES

<u>**CONDITION OVERVIEW**</u>:
Arteries are the largest blood vessels that carry oxygen-rich blood from the heart to various parts of the body. Veins are thinner vessels that carry blood back towards the heart while Capillaries are the smallest of all blood vessels. Capillaries are so small, that sometimes only a few red blood cells can pass through the center of the capillary at a time, so...if you have to see bleeding on your beloved pet, you should hope for Capillary Bleeding. They connect arteries to veins and near the surface can be found in the mucus membranes (gums, eye lids, ears and surface). Most of the time capillaries ooze rather than bleed, and mostly require superficial cleaning, antibiotic ointment and maybe a bandage to keep dirt and infection at bay.

From an artery, blood spurts as it is coming directly from the pump...the heart. It will be bright red in color since it is well-oxygenated coming from the lungs and there may be a lot of it! Controlling blood loss, bandaging to prevent infection and getting veterinary treatment all need to be accomplished quickly.

Since veins too are large vessels, much blood loss can occur. Generally, the blood is a little darker in color as it has given up oxygen on its return route to the lungs and has picked up toxins along the way. The blood will pool rather than spurt as it is not feeling the pressure of the heart pump, but same protocol is in order as for an artery...control bleeding, bandage to prevent infection and quick veterinary attention.

<u>**PREVENTIVE MEASURES/CAUSES**</u>:
- Get down on all fours in your house and yard and watch for sharp items that could cut a paw, catch on an ear or tail or poke an eye. Additionally, with our feline friends you must pay attention to sharp edges on counter tops and shelving if they are prone to jump up.
- Keep nails well-trimmed as a long nail can break and cause severe bleeding.
- Keep cats indoors to avoid fights (and therefore puncture wounds) with other animals and to prevent pets from being hit by cars. Make sure ears, tails and other body parts don't get squeezed in doors (house or car).

<u>**SIGNS & SYMPTOMS**</u>:
- Appearance of blood whether it's oozing, pooling or spurting.
- If blood appears under the skin like a pocket or sack, this is called a Hematoma and requires a veterinary aspiration of the blood. If delayed, surgery may be required. Most commonly occurs in floppy ears that are scratched or bang a wall or table when a kitty shakes their head.

WHAT YOU MAY NEED:
- 4 X 4 Gauze Squares
- Gauze Roll
- Blunt-Nosed Scissors to cut bandage materials as well as trim fur around wound
- Purified Water, Eye Wash (saline), Antibacterial soap, Chlorhexidine
- Antibacterial cream or gel (Neosporin®-like product) or pure aloe vera gel
- Towels, phone book or pillow to elevate injured areas higher than the pet's heart
- Miscellaneous old socks, pieces of panty hose, t-shirts, children's garments to help secure bandage around head, chest or tail

WHAT TO DO:
For minor cuts and scrapes:

Trim fur with blunt-nosed scissors to reveal wound.

Flush with water, saline solution, eye wash, antibacterial soap or Chlorhexidine (Hibiclens®)

Pat dry and apply antibacterial ointment or pure aloe vera gel to promote healing. Apply just enough to cover wound so that it will soak in, not leaving excess to be licked off.

If cat starts to lick wound, bandage (see page 122) or apply a cone collar to prevent pet from getting to injury. Using the self-adhering wrap that contains an anti-lick taste often helps. Try it yourself, it's icky LOL

For bleeding toe nails, pour dime to quarter-sized amount of styptic powder into the palm of your hand and press bleeding toe nail into the powder, also applying direct pressure against your palm until the bleeding stops. Watch for any signs of infection (redness, swelling, oozing or heat).

For severe bleeding injuries to the legs or limbs there are 3 courses of action to be taken to stop bleeding and promote clotting:

1) Apply direct pressure with gauze squares directly over the wound. If that alone doesn't stop the bleeding...

2) Elevate the limb by placing a pillow or folded towel underneath the injured body part keeping it higher than the animal's heart. If you still need help getting the bleeding to stop...

3) Apply pressure to one of 5 pressure points on your cat. Pressure points are arteries located closest to the surface of the skin, so applying pressure on the one corresponding to the injury, will lessen blood loss. (Think of a straw...if it's fully open, you can get the good stuff through, but if you squeeze it flatter, less will flow. The same applies to blood and oxygen travelling through your pet's blood vessels.)

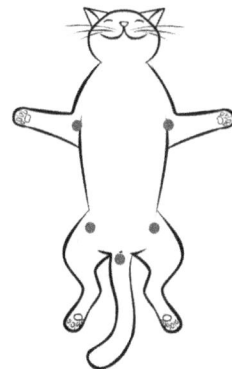

Image Courtesy of Sunny-dog Ink

FRONT LEG (Brachial Artery) – Place your thumb on the outside of the upper leg and your fingers on the inside close to the armpit to reduce blood flow and allow clotting to occur.

HIND LEG (Femoral Artery) – Turn pet on his back or side if possible, place two fingers at the stifle or knee and slide your fingers into the upper fleshy thigh near where his leg meets his groin. Press.

TAIL (Caudal Artery) – Steady your kitty by holding her against your chest against you (head towards your rear) with one arm her back and around her belly. With your other hand, lift the tail and apply pressure firmly with your thumb on top of the tail (at the base where it meets the body) and two or three fingers underneath the tail.

Once bleeding stops, wrap flat gauze with rolled gauze, overlapping each layer by about ¾ widths each time around the leg, then secure with self-adhering elastic bandage making sure you can slip a finger underneath so as not to cut off circulation, then get professional medical help.

NOTE: Be patient. Realize stopping bleeding could take 5 - 10 minutes, however if excessive blood loss is occurring, do your best to keep direct pressure and quickly transport animal to nearest veterinary office. If the bandage is too tight, it's unlikely you'll see skin turning blue, as in humans. With pets, you are more likely to notice swelling above or below the bandage if it is too tight, or coolness to the skin below the bandage (as it is not receiving sufficient blood flow). Stay alert and loosen if you observe either.

BANDAGING TIP: After gauze is securely covered, just once take the gauze roll around the lower abdomen (when bandaging a hind leg) or once around the chest for the front leg, and then back around wound area. This creates "suspenders" -- a method to hold the bandage up. Legs are like vertical poles, and if the bandage is only wrapped around the leg, it can slide down once the cat stands.

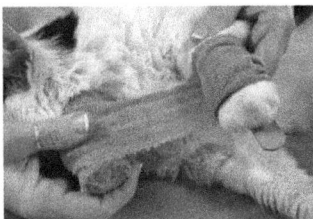

Photo by: Sunny-dog Ink

Never apply a tourniquet to control severe bleeding unless it's the only way to save a life, knowing that the paw or leg below the tourniquet will probably require amputation.

NOTE: In a situation where bleeding is profuse, if all you have is a clean towel, apply that to the wound and with someone else driving, continue to hold the towel and get the cat as quickly as possible to the Veterinarian. It's always wise to call ahead so that Veterinarian technicians can be ready to assist you.

Paw Pad Wounds
- Remove obvious debris and flush to clean if it's oozing, but if bleeding profusely, stop blood loss.
- Elevate to aid direct pressure and/or apply pressure to appropriate pressure point.
- Wrap paw with gauze encircling pad, and then between each of the toes - in a figure eight pattern - to hold it in place.

- Secure firmly but not tight with self-adhering wrap. The self-adhering wrap has texture and will provide traction.
- An alternative would be to slip a human sock over the bandage to keep it in place.

After treatment at your Veterinarian's office, you will be told to keep bandaging dry.

Ear Injuries
- For direct pressure... Apply gauze square to bleeding and then press "upright" ears down towards the side of the face or check.
- Ears are higher than heart so you have built-in elevation!
- No pressure on arteries as we don't want to cut off blood to the brain.
- Bandage in place using the good ear as an anchor (go around front of good ear first, then behind) to secure in place. If you just go around the front of the good ear with each pass, the bandage will fall down the face; if you just go behind the good ear, the bandage will fall down the neck. Obviously, do your best not to cover the cat's eyes or cause pressure to the throat when bandaging his head.
- A helpful final step is to use the sleeve off a cotton t-shirt or cut the toe off a cotton sock or thigh out of panty hose (depending on the size of the pet's head) and use as a "headband" over the ears to hold bandage in place.
- For small nicks or cuts to the ear, styptic powder may be used to control bleeding, but never use styptic powder on a deep or large wound.

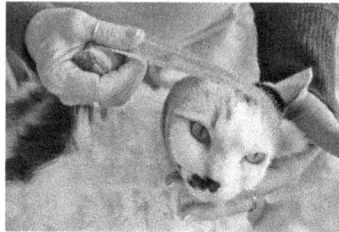

Photo by: Sunny-dog Ink

Tail Injuries
- Apply direct pressure with gauze pad to tail wound, and lift tail to elevate.
- If needed, press on pressure point (Caudal Artery) at base of tail (where tail meets body) to diminish blood flow.
- Wrap tail with gauze roll to secure flat pad, then slip a child's-size cotton tube sock or leotard leg over the gauze roll.
- To further secure, if you deem necessary, beginning at tip of tail, wrap sock in a criss-cross pattern with adhesive tape going up the tail and 2" beyond sock and directly onto fur.
- Complete by criss-crossing back down the tail being careful not to wrap too tightly.

Chest Injuries
- Apply direct pressure with a flat square of gauze directly over the wound.
- There are no applicable pressure points as many blood vessels cross this area of the body.
- When applying gauze roll, wrap it around entire torso to hold in place then secure it to itself with adhesive tape. Consider only going around chest twice and then taping remaining roll of gauze onto wound to apply more direct pressure and create absorbency should wound re-start bleeding enroute to veterinary assistance.
- You can doubly secure by placing a triangular bandage under pet's chest on top of bandage and knot at back/shoulders to hold in place.
- An alternative is to fit the pet with a baby's cotton t-shirt on top of the bandage or once again, depending on size of the animal, using the thigh out of panty hose, sleeve off adult t-shirt or whatever makes a snug covering. Not too tight though to limit breathing!

Important Note:

If bleeding does not stop within 5-10 minutes after applying direct pressure, seek veterinary care immediately.

BITES & STINGS

One Summer morning, Scottish Fold kittens were playfully exploring their fenced yard when Ruby caught Abigail off guard and bounded at her from behind the rose bushes. As Abby took a tumble landing dazed and confused, a bumble bee buzzed passed her. The twosome, quickly distracted by this new found fun, attempted to play a game of pounce with the tiny buzzing creature. Fun did ensue for a few moments, but it then turned nasty as the bee planted his stinger right onto the tip of Ruby's nose! The kitty pawed furiously at her face, and as it began to swell, Ruby started looking more like a Bulldog than a kitty cat.

CONDITION OVERVIEW:
Cats are natural hunters and often go in search of smaller critters as prey. Just as with humans, our pets can experience an allergic or inflammatory reaction if bitten or stung. Most pets, are bitten or stung on the face or in the mouth since they snap at bees and other insects. Sometimes they are even stung inside their mouth but can also sit or step on a stinging insect.

PREVENTIVE MEASURES/CAUSES:
- Do your best to lessen the prey drive in your pet (using the word "no" or having a water squirt bottle nearby to deter their desire to participate in the chase), but nature will unfortunately take its course, so be prepared when the inevitable happens.

- Keep down the insect population by not leaving food outside, using pet-safe insecticides around your yard and growing plants (such as lemongrass or catnip - Your cat will love this!) or lighting citronella candles (if safe around pets) that cause insects to stay away.

SIGNS & SYMPTOMS:
- Swelling
- Pawing at face or licking paws or site of sting
- Breathing difficulty -- AN EMERGENCY SITUATION

Important Note:

Anaphylactic Shock - Some animals, like people, are highly sensitive to insect toxin and can go into Anaphylactic Shock (a severe allergic reaction which can cause the circulatory system to shut down). If you notice any of the following symptoms, which usually occur within one hour, you must seek veterinary assistance immediately:

1) Severe and profuse swelling (i.e. entire face as opposed to just the lip)
2) Difficulty breathing or increased respiratory effort possibly due to swelling of the tongue or throat.
3) Vomiting & Diarrhea
4) Very pale or blue-tinged mucous membranes (cyanosis)
5) Rapid and/or irregular pulse
6) Prolonged CRT (Capillary Refill Time) - Refer to 5 Vital Checks - pages 92-97
7) Below normal body temperature (less than 100° F)

WHAT YOU MAY NEED:
- Cold Pack
- Baking Soda or Meat Tenderizer Containing Papain.
- Epi-pen (if your pet has had previous encounters with bees and is allergic)
- Water
- Needle-less Syringe
- Eye Dropper
- Spray Bottle
- Diphenhydramine/Benadryl® (not containing Cetirizine, Acetaphetamine or Pseudoephedrine)

NOTE: If you can find liquid gel caps, pierce the cap with a straight pin and administer medicine by squirting liquid from the cap underneath the pet's tongue. The abundance of blood vessels in the mouth allows the medicine to be absorbed more quickly into the blood stream sublingually than if swallowed and processed by the stomach.

WHAT TO DO:

INSECT STINGS (Bees/Wasps):

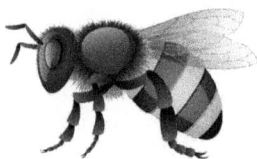

If you see the stinger, flick it away with a credit card, popsicle stick or even your finger nail. Do not pull the stinger with your fingers or tweezers as you are likely to puncture the poison sac allowing the toxin to enter your cat's body. Often though there is no stinger to be found as it is concealed in the pet's fur or has already been pawed away.

Administer 1 mg Diphenhydramine (Benadryl® antihistamine) for every pound your pet weighs (ex: 60 lbs. dog needs 60 mg). Although this medication is generally safe, check with your Veterinarian especially if your pet is taking other medications or has any known medical conditions. It will make the animal sleepy and hopefully prevent him from further scratching. Diphenhydramine should not contain cetirizine, acetaphenomine or pseudoephedrine. This dose can be repeated in 6-8 hours if swelling persists. Beyond that, seek veterinary care.

Apply cold pack to any swelling, but remove every few minutes to avoid frostbite. You can also squeeze out a wet washcloth till it is just damp and place it between cold pack and kitty to dissipate coldness.

Should you actually be able to see through your pet's fur and locate the sting site, dab it with a paste made of 1 Tablespoon baking soda or meat tenderizer mixed with a drop of water to counteract the acidity of the toxin (meat tenderizer and baking soda are alkaline). The tenderizer contains papain, an enzyme extract from papayas which breaks down the protein in the toxin. Diphenhydramine should not contain cetirizine, acetophenomine or pseudoephedrine. Baking soda and meat tenderizer also work for fire ant and jelly fish stings but not against snake venom while white vinegar is best for wasp stings.

If you have an epi-pen prescribed specifically for your cat, read attached instructions but inject one dose and get to your Veterinarian as when the epinephrine wears off, anaphylaxis can occur.

HOMEOPATHIC TIP:

Apis Meliffica, can aid the body to reduce burning or stinging pain. A dose is considered to be 3-5 pellets crushed or liquefied with 6c being given every 4-6 hours.

IF INSECT STING IS IN THE MOUTH:

- Offer pet an ice cube, frozen slice of banana or ice water to minimize swelling.
- Seek immediate advice from your veterinary professional as toxins in the mucous membranes of the mouth and under the tongue more quickly absorb into the cat's blood stream and should his tongue swell, a Veterinarian is best equipped to help.
- Call your Veterinarian as you are on the way to find out if you should administer 1mg Diphenhydramine for every pound the pet weighs or if you should wait till you arrive at the Animal Hospital.

SCORPIONS

From human experience, we know the pain from a scorpion sting can be intense. When stung, most pets recover without difficulty, however some do have a more severe reaction. There are over 1,200 different species of scorpions in the world and their venom varies with most potent enough to kill an insect or small animals, but some deadly to larger animals and humans. Scorpions can control the amount of venom injected, and those with large thick tails and slender pinchers are generally more harmful.

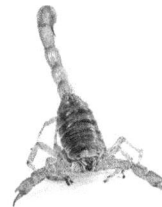

Contrary to some beliefs, cats are not immune to a scorpion's sting. They generally notice scorpions and do not step on them like dogs or humans might and are more agile and faster so often avoid the sting altogether.

PREVENTIVE MEASURES/CAUSES:
- Do not allow cats to roam in areas that are known to have venomous scorpions. Especially when temperatures climb above 100°F, Scorpions like damp areas around wood piles, flower beds with wood chips and plumbing fixtures, so make sure your kitty can't access these areas.
- Deter scorpions from entering your home by repairing holes in window screens and adding weather stripping and caulk to seal any holes scorpions might enter through.
- Prune trees and shrubbery from near the house.
- The use of cedar oil may repel scorpions or if a problem, investigate pet-safe insecticides.

SIGNS & SYMPTOMS:
- Localized pain and/or numbness, But more severe include:
  - Drooling
  - Tearing from the eyes
  - Inappropriate urination and defecation (loss of control of bodily functions)
  - Dilated pupils
  - Muscle tremors
  - Breathing difficulty
  - Collapse

WHAT YOU MAY NEED:
- A calm you to transport your pet to the Veterinarian for assessment.
- Dead scorpion for identification if you can obtain safely.

WHAT TO DO:
Carefully remove the stinger from your pet if at all possible, but prompt veterinary care is strongly recommended where supportive treatment (fluids and pain medications) will be provided.

SPIDERS

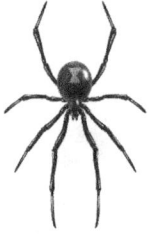

With over 30,000 species in the world, spiders exist everywhere! Most spider bites however cause little more than painful swelling and should be treated like bee or wasp stings since most spiders are unable to penetrate human or animal skin. There are a few species in the U.S. however, and more throughout the world that are venomous (inject toxin through fangs) and in addition to inflicting a painful bite, can cause our pets to experience serious side effects within 30 minutes to several hours of being stung. Cats tend to get multiple bites due to their tendency to poke at and harass the spider.

In the United States, these include: Widow (5 species), Brown Recluse and Hobo spiders. The most dangerous arachnids around the world include: Brazilian Wandering, Six-Eyed Sand, Sidney Funnel Web, Redback, Mouse and Yellow Sac spiders. If your pet is bitten by one of these, get immediate veterinary help!

PREVENTIVE MEASURES/CAUSES:
- Use pet-safe insecticides to keep your house and yard spider-free.
- Clear debris piles and leaves from locations your pets hang out.
- Prevent cats from sniffing under and around sheds, foundations, basements and damp areas, including where hoses are stored, near water spigots and leaky plumbing -- basically cool, dark, damp locations.

SIGNS & SYMPTOMS:
- Swelling/Redness
- Licking at or rubbing area of the sting
- In severe cases...pain, fever, rash, chills, breathing difficulty, vomiting, diarrhea, lethargy, muscle tremors or rigidness, paralysis (including of the lungs) and Shock

WHAT YOU MAY NEED:
- Benadryl® (not containing Cetirizine, Acetaphetamine or Pseudoephedrine)
- Baking Soda or Meat Tenderizer
- Water
- Cold Pack

WHAT TO DO:
As in Bee Stings already discussed, Administer 1 mg Diphenhydramine (Benadryl® antihistamine) for every pound your pet weighs (ex: 10 lbs. cat needs 10 mg). Benadryl® should not contain cetirizine, acetaphenomine or pseudoephedrine and do not give cats time release capsules. See Allergy page 113 for more details. Spider toxin also contains acid, so applying an alkaline baking soda or meat tenderizer paste (as described in BEE STINGS) may counteract the acidity.

Apply cold pack to any swelling, but remove every few minutes to avoid frostbite.

If you suspect your cat has been bitten by a venomous spider, apply a cold pack, restrain his movement (movement hastens the spread of venom) and get him quickly to your Veterinarian. If you can, bring the dead spider with you unless you already know what kind of spider it was.

Black Widow Spiders terrify us all with their distinctive red hour-glass marking (some are brown with orange hour glasses, mostly in Florida but they travel). About ½" - 1" long (1.2cm - 2.54 cm) they prefer warm, dry climates and spin their webs in crevices and protected dark locations. Both the male and female Black Widow possess a nerve toxin, but only the female has long enough fangs to penetrate a pet's skin. If you could find the bite under the animal's fur, you may note a slight redness with two small puncture wounds 1-2mm apart. Muscle cramps, pain, increased heart rate, vomiting, diarrhea and paralysis follow. Cats may experience more severe effects due to the venom ratio to their smaller body size, but location of the bite, health and age of the pet and even time of the year (venom is thought to be more potent during warmer times of year) all play a role. If you suspect a bite, have your Veterinarian evaluate your pet immediately. Antivenin is available with mixed results but pain medications and muscle relaxants may help pull your pet through.

Brown Recluse (aka Fiddleback) Spiders tend to hide in dark, secluded areas and their venom is known to destroy tissue (necrosis) surrounding the bite. Approximately ½" - 2" long (1.2cm - 5cm), the Brown Recluse can be identified by a distinctive fiddle-shaped mark on its back. Generally found in the South Central U.S. (Texas through Georgia) they are being found elsewhere. When bitten, some pets do not realize it, but after a while redness occurs often in the shape of a bulls-eye which is generally not noticeable on our pets. Seek veterinary assistance at once. Animals are treated with pain medications and antibiotics and some wounds require surgical closure.

Hobo or Travelling Spiders can destroy your pet's tissue with their bite. Found mostly in the Pacific Northwest, these large and aggressive brown spiders (often confused with the Recluse) build their webs in basements or at ground level. If a bite is suspected, get your pet to the Veterinarian!

Many **Tarantulas** are furry exotic pets but some species found in the U.S. produce venom that can cause localized pain. Not only can the mild venom cause problems for your cat or dog, but also the ingestion of the stiff hair covering the spider's legs can cause irritation to your pet's mouth including pain, drooling and vomiting. Tarantula's can actually "flick" hairs at targets when threatened, so don't allow pet's to get too close. If your pet is bitten, no serious problems should be expected but it is always best to err on the side of caution and have your Veterinarian check Fluffy out. On the reverse...the jumping nature of your eight-legged pet Tarantula makes it an irresistible plaything to many four-legged pets, and a Tarantula can die from a bite caused by a cat.

CONDITION OVERVIEW:

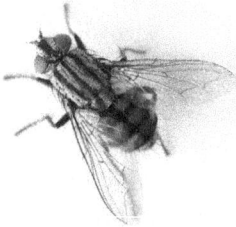

Cats with upright ears seem to hold the biggest temptation for flies but the bridge of the nose or any body part where skin is visible can be bitten. The Stable Fly – which looks like a regular House Fly – has bayonet-like, needle-sharp mouthparts which it uses to get blood from your pet. Cats with fly bites don't bleed much but the ear tips get crusty from inflammation and the serum that leaks from the bites. Fly bites leave bloody lumps on your pet and in the worst cases, lay eggs from which maggots can hatch.

PREVENTIVE MEASURES/CAUSES:

- Remove items that attract flies: pick up pet feces daily, cover garbage cans, pick up fallen fruit
- Place fly traps in strategic locations if this is a serious problem
- Bring your dog inside, especially during warm weather when flies congregate most
- Apply petroleum jelly or Avon® Skin-so-Soft lotion on the tips of your pet's ears to deter flies
- Add 1 Tablespoon Apple Cider Vinegar to your cat's water -- some people swear flies won't bite an animal or human who drinks Apple Cider Vinegar!

WHAT YOU MAY NEED:

- Chlorhexidine or mild soap
- Triple Antibiotic Cream (Neosporin®-type product)
- Warm, wet washcloth or gauze squares

WHAT TO DO:

Soften the scab with a warm wet washcloth. Take 2-3 minutes until it can be gently wiped away.

Clean with plain warm water.

Apply an antibiotic ointment to prevent infection and keep your pets fly-free.

If your cat must be outside, consult with your Veterinarian in regards to a topical fly repellant that can be applied to your animal.

If wounds won't heal or you see any presence of maggots, get your pet to professional veterinary help!

SNAKES

CONDITION OVERVIEW:

Another danger to our pets comes in the form of venomous and non-venomous snakes. Yes, even those without venom (toxic saliva) carry bacteria in their mouths (they don't brush their teeth and consume rats and mice on a daily basis) which can cause infection in your pet. The physical appearance of each snake species varies, and it may be difficult to tell which species you've encountered unless you are familiar with herpetology (the study of amphibians and reptiles).

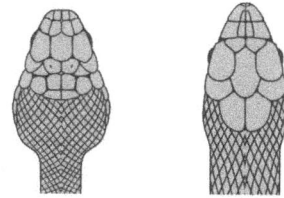

Here are general guidelines to help you determine if what you are seeing is a poisonous snake although there are always exceptions to the rule:

- A broad, triangular head with a noticeable "neck"
- Elliptical pupils (vertical slits) like cats for pupils while non-venomous snakes generally have round pupils like us and our dogs (hopefully you won't be close enough to evaluate this!)
- "Pit vipers" have heat-sensing "pits" (thermo-receptors) on their faces between the eye and nostril which help them locate prey, especially warm-blooded animals.
- Two fangs which leave puncture wounds. Non-venomous snakes leave a bite or bruise mark that resembles a row of teeth – like when you bite out of a sandwich but much smaller.
- In the case of the rattlesnake, a rattle is present which may or may not issue a warning.

Rattles are made of keratin, similar to our fingernails. When a baby snake is born, he has one button/segment of his rattle. Each time he sheds his skin, he acquires another segment (shedding typically occurs several times a year based on food supply and growth). At least two segments are required to vibrate against each other to create a noise. If a snake has not shed his skin for the first time he will not be able to rattle. Snakes generally carry their rattles high to protect them, they do break from time to time. Although rattles are considered warning devices, some snakes have evolved into not using them as the sound wards off prey that could become a tasty meal.

Venomous snakes can be found in rural areas as well as suburban areas where there is sufficient natural habitat. In cold climates most hibernate from November through March. In warmer climates, however they are active year round, and after mild winters, they come out of hibernation early.

Follow the WHAT TO DO steps below for any of these venomous snakes and get your pet to the Veterinarian immediately!

- Rattlesnakes can be found throughout most of the south from California to Florida.
- Copperheads live mostly in North Florida to Massachusetts and westward to Texas and Nebraska.
- Cottonmouths/Water moccasins inhabit Illinois, Missouri, Oklahoma and Texas north east to Virginia and south to Florida.
- Coral snakes are typically found in the Southeast (Texas to Florida) and have tri-colored bands of red, yellow and black that completely encircle the body. "Red touching yellow is a dangerous fellow" as opposed to the "red touching black, venom he lacks" scarlet king snake which is non-venomous. King snakes in other parts of the country are colored differently.

Learn which species are indigenous to your neighborhood as well as to any locations you may travel to with your pet. The list above is only a guideline, so just like you must know your cat, you need to know what local dangers she may encounter BEFORE she does so!

Most snakes can control the amount of venom they inject and often deliver a "dry" bite to a human or large animal. Baby snakes, however, are born with venom and the means to inject it but aren't yet "fang trained," so generally hold on longer and deliver all the venom they have at one time. Older snakes possess more potent venom and larger snakes store larger volumes of it.

This toxic fluid, made from up to 25 different enzymes, comes in two forms created in specialized oral glands: Hemotoxic venom disrupts the integrity of the blood vessels causing swelling as blood seeps into the tissue and prevents clotting. It also breaks down the tissue and "pre-digests" it making it easier for the snake to consume. Neurotoxic venom results in paralysis including that of the respiratory muscles ending in suffocation. Some snakes possess both types.

The degree of severity of any venomous snake bite depends on several factors:
- The species & size of snake
- The size of the animal bitten
- The amount of venom injected (approximately 20% of bites are "dry" meaning envenomation has not occurred, but that means 80% of the time it has!)

PREVENTIVE MEASURES/CAUSES:
- As with many other scenarios requiring pet first-aid, prevention is key, so your best safety device is keeping control of the animals in your care. It is easier to prevent snake bites than it is to treat them.
- Eliminate garbage, wood piles and even ivy from pet play areas. These are favorite locales of mice, and where mice hang out…snakes line up for dinner!

SIGNS & SYMPTOMS:

- Puncture wounds ("U" shaped bite or bruise if non-venomous)
- Drooling
- Shortness of breath
- Swelling
- Diarrhea
- Seizures/convulsions
- Inability to bark
- Paralysis
- Shock

WHAT YOU MAY NEED:

- As in most pet first-aid…a calm you! Phone and phone number to call ahead
- Transportation to the Animal ER
- Chlorhexidine/antibacterial soap ONLY if a non-venomous bite

WHAT TO DO:
If you are certain it was a <u>non-venomous</u> snake…

Wash the wound with antibacterial soap and observe.

If red or warm to the touch, get to the Veterinarian for antibiotics or other treatment.

If an animal in your care is bitten by a snake, it is best to assume it was a <u>venomous</u> bite and proceed as follows:

- Keep bite wound below level of heart to prevent speedy absorption to heart.
- Keep kitty calm – the faster he moves, the faster the venom circulates.
- Get the animal to an emergency veterinary hospital immediately to be sure they have antivenin. Treatment should begin within 30 minutes of the bite, and it takes 30 minutes to mix the antidote!

WHAT NOT TO DO:

- **Do NOT** cut over the bite and try to suck out the poison. You will not be successful and may absorb under your tongue or in any mouth sore. Additionally by cutting tissue, you are more readily allowing toxin to be absorbed.
- **Do NOT** manipulate the bitten area or allow the pet to move about freely.
- **Do NOT** place an ice pack over the bite. This will concentrate the toxin more locally causing extensive, irreparable tissue damage.

Important Note:
Antivenin is an antidote: a serum produced to neutralize the effects of the venom. In laboratories, healthy horses are injected with increasing amounts (non-fatal) of selected snake venom causing the horse to create antibodies from which the antivenin is made. A specific antibody is produced for each type of snake (typically four different crotaline/rattlesnakes). Antivenin is reconstituted before use and given to your furry patient

via an IV drip that takes 30+ minutes per vial. It is expensive ($800 - $1,500 per vial) and although a large dog is likely to require 3-4 vials, some many require up to 10 vials to save their lives, plus antibiotics, fluids and pain medications to see him through. Antivenin is only currently available for certain species of snakes. Pets bitten by other species are treated for symptoms presented. This just underscores the importance of avoidance training and diligent supervision if you frequent or live in areas that are common for venomous snakes.

Rattlesnake Vaccine is not a cure-all but can minimize the severity, which has the two-fold benefit of giving more time (before death occurs) to get to a Veterinarian and may reduce the number of antivenin vials needed for treatment. For these reasons, the vaccination is beneficial if you live in a snake-prone area. Check with your Veterinarian for details and if it is advised for cats in your area..

Jelly Fish Stings

CONDITION OVERVIEW:

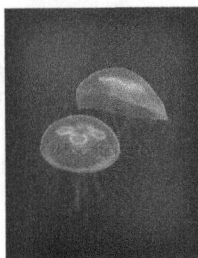

It is the rare cat that roams the shore, but in the event you know one… Jelly fish are extraordinary yet simple marine animals characterized by their jelly-like bodies and stinging tentacles. Among the oldest creatures on earth, there are around 10,000 different species and they get their proper name "cnidarians" from the Greek word for "sea nettle." When they come in contact with prey -- meaning you or your cat – their tentacles literally explode causing great pain

PREVENTIVE MEASURES/CAUSES:

Avoid high risk areas when visiting the beach with your sea faring feline by:
- Looking for warning signs – diamond shape informational signs that depict a human and a jelly fish.
- Noticing purple flags which denote dangerous marine life.
- Keep your cat away from the water's edge during windy times. Jelly fish come near shore when it is windy and show up in large numbers (known as blooms).
- Do not touch or let your cat anywhere near a jelly fish, even if it appears dead. Poisonous cells on dead jelly fish can still sting! They often look like plastic bags, bluish-purple bottles or light bulbs. Keep a watchful eye and keep your kitty out of harm's way.

WHAT YOU MAY NEED:
- Rubbing alcohol or white vinegar
- Rubber Gloves
- Stick tape - any kind but NOT duct tape
- Benadryl® (not containing Cetirizine, Acetaphetamine or Pseudoephedrine)
- Baking Soda
- Ice pack

WHAT TO DO:

Put on rubber gloves or you will be stung too, and pour rubbing alcohol or white vinegar onto the tentacles. This stabilizes the namtocysts preventing them from continuing to sting your pet. Next take small sections of sticky tape (like for packing boxes) and gently press against tentacle, pull tape away to remove. Once you've done a good clean-up of the tentacles, flush the affected area with salt water or even beach sand. Fresh water will cause toxins to be released into your pet! Call your Veterinarian and you may be advised to administer Benedryl® (1mg per pound of your pet's body weight). Packing the site of the sting with a baking soda/water paste may soothe the pain as can a cold compress. After 10 - 20 minutes, alternate every 5 minutes with a very warm (but not scalding) towel. Remove and let it cool to bring healing blood back to the area flushing out the toxin. Then reapply the cold compress followed by the warm towel for about 20 minutes or until veterinary care is reached.

BLOOD SUGAR ISSUES -

Low (Hypoglycemia or Fading) & High (Hyperglycemia/Diabetes Mellitus)

CONDITION OVERVIEW:

Insulin, a hormone that is produced and released by the pancreas into the bloodstream when glucose levels rise, plays a key role in maintaining normal sugar levels. As it moves glucose through the body, it gives ours pets their energy for life. The normal blood sugar level for cats is 75 to 120 mg/dl (milligrams per deciliter), but the level can be as high as 250 to 300 mg/dl after a meal or in stressful situations, such as visiting the Veterinarian's office.

Hypoglycemia (aka low blood sugar) occurs when levels drop below 60 mg/dl. It primarily occurs in our tiniest four-legged friends, including Toy breeds and juvenile animals (less than 4 months of age). Very active adult dogs, however, may experience low sugar if sustained exercise has caused a depletion in liver glycogen (sugar).

When not enough insulin is produced hyperglycemia is the outcome and your cat may be diagnosed with diabetes mellitus if sugar levels exceed 400mg/dl. This means conscientious pet parenting is a must as a lifetime of treatment is in store for your cat, starting with insulin injections and a special diet to keep the sugars in check.

PREVENTIVE MEASURES/CAUSES FOR HYPOGLYCEMIA (low blood sugar):

- Annual check-ups and blood tests as suggested by your Veterinarian can alert you to a problem.
- Susceptible kitties should be fed small amounts frequently throughout the day of a high quality protein and fiber/low sugar, carbohydrate and fat diet as instructed by your Veterinarian. This will help keep glucose levels constant. Also, check if adding a tablespoon of Karo® Syrup to your pet's daily drinking water would be beneficial for at-risk pets. If you do so though, you MUST change the water EVERY day as the sugar can grow bacteria (You are however changing the water and washing the bowl daily anyway with warm soapy water, right? It's an important part of good cat parenting!).

- Extremely active pets should receive high quality protein before exhibiting long bouts of energy, but of course with a lengthy digestion period in between to prevent bloat..
- Keep any product containing xylitol out of pawsand claws reach as it causes an increase in insulin which can drop your pet's glucose level in 30 minutes to 12 hours after ingestion. Read labels on sugar-free sweeteners, gums and candies, certain jams and baking products, over–the–counter and prescription medications and dental hygiene products as well as anything you suspect your pet could ingest that could contain xylitol or anything labeled "sugar alcohols". Veterinary treatment is key as liver failure can result.

SIGNS & SYMPTOMS FOR HYPOGLYCEMIA (low blood sugar):
- Twitching, shaking or wooziness; disorientation as if they are intoxicated
- Weakness/lethargy
- Head tilt
- Seizures
- Loss of consciousness

This is serious. Pets can die without quick first-aid and medical attention if diabetic!

WHAT YOU MAY NEED FOR HYPOGLYCEMIA (low blood sugar):
- Karo® or Pancake Syrup
- Honey
- Needle-less Syringe or Eye Dropper
- Blanket

WHAT TO DO FOR HYPOGLYCEMIA (low blood sugar):
The quickest way to reverse hypoglycemia is to administer sugar by mouth (honey, Karo Syrup®, pancake syrup) –
  1 teaspoon for pets under 50 lbs.
  2 teaspoons for animals 50 - 80 lbs.
  2 ½ - 3 teaspoons for extra-large breeds.

If cat is unconscious or can't swallow, rub the syrup on the lips and gums. If cat is not alert and breathing normally, treat for shock (See page 188 to increase circulation and cover to keep in body heat) as you seek immediate veterinary attention. Watch for breathing and check for pulse and administer rescue breathing and/or CPR if needed.

PREVENTIVE MEASURES/CAUSES FOR HYPERGLYCEMIA (high blood sugar):
- Avoid high intake of sugar in your cat's diet.
- Don't miss annual check-ups or let infections go unchecked.

SIGNS & SYMPTOMS FOR HYPERGLYCEMIA (high blood sugar):
- Increased thirst and/or hunger
- Increased urination
- Weight loss or weight gain
- Dehydration
- Cataracts and/or inflamed blood vessels in the eyes
- Enlarged Liver
- Open sores that won't heal
- Nerve damage in limbs

WHAT YOU MAY NEED FOR HYPERGLYCEMIA (high blood sugar):
- Prescribed medication and syringe (see page 100 for details on giving injections, but learning in person from your Veterinarian is best).

WHAT TO DO FOR HYPERGLYCEMIA (high blood sugar):
Once diagnosed, diabetic cats can live a wonderful life with human caretakers as long as life-long compliance is maintained to properly manage the disease. Urine and ear prick testing with an at-home glucometer can help keep your Fluffy's glucose levels in check.

If insulin has been prescribed, correct dosing is a must at the right time of day. Too much, not enough or a too soon or delayed dose can be very dangerous for your furry friend. Additionally, a special low sugar and low carbohydrate diet with higher protein and fiber may be recommended. It is imperative that you strictly follow treatment guidelines for the health of your canine or feline patient and friend.

BURNS

CONDITION OVERVIEW:
Just like in humans, the skin is your dog or cat's largest organ, and serious injury can happen to it. Heat, chemicals and electrical sources can all be the cause. Second and third degree burns are highly susceptible to infection since many layers of tissue have been destroyed. A visit to your Veterinarian is in order, but cooling the skin is essential and should be done slowly over a 30 minute period.

PREVENTIVE MEASURES/CAUSES:
- Be aware of ever-present dangers...when you have a cat, you have an inquisitive furry toddler for life.
- Cats love heat and will lounge on surfaces well over 100° F; this includes your oven, stove and clothes dryer.
- Beware when removing pots and pans from still-hot burners by preventing Fluffy from jumping up, and never pass hot plates or liquids over your pet's head. Also, think twice about stepping over pets, especially with anything in your hands, as it is Murphy's Law that when you step over your pet will move and trip you!
- Candles, even on countertops, can be toppled by or burn cats who jump up high.

- Supervise pets around fire pits/camp fires, fireplaces and heat sources of all types -- electric heaters, furnaces, hot pavement, even beach sand during the peak of summer.
- Too much sun can burn the muzzle, ear tips, back or belly. A shorter summer trim is fine but never shave your pet as fur protects his skin from the harsh sun.
- Beach sand, sidewalks and asphalt can burn paws…if you can't walk on it barefoot, it's too hot for your outdoor cat!
- Anything hot to the touch -- if you could get burned, so could your cat!

First Degree Burns

SIGNS & SYMPTOMS:
Skin appears pink to dark pink or red (usually sunburn on the snout, ears or belly skin), could be slightly swollen

WHAT YOU MAY NEED:
- Room Temperature Water
- Cold Pack
- Aloe Vera Gel or Triple Anti-biotic Cream
- Soft Cloth or Gauze
- Blunt-Nosed Scissors

NOTE: Thermal burns start out sterile as heat kills bacteria. Take care not to contaminate wounds by trying to "clean" or cover with non-sterile materials.

WHAT TO DO:
The first goal is to cool the pink skin with room temperature water (not ice water which restricts circulation).

Pat dry and apply pure aloe vera gel to promote healing after carefully trimming fur away with blunt-nosed scissors.

If skin is unbroken, home care should suffice by holding a cold pack (not ice) over the wound for another 20 minutes and observing that it heals while preventing your pet from obsessive licking or scratching the injured area.

Second Degree Burns

SIGNS & SYMPTOMS:
- Pink to red skin with the presence of blisters and/or serous fluid (aka pus)
- Extremely painful & susceptible to infection as tissue damage has occurred

WHAT YOU MAY NEED:
- Muzzle
- Room Temperature Water
- Soft Cloth
- Non-stick/Teflon Coated Gauze Pad
- Gauze Roll or Clean White Sheet to Cover
- Adhesive Tape to Secure Loose Bandage

WHAT TO DO:

Get to your Veterinarian but call first! Intravenous fluids, antibiotics and hospitalization may be needed.

Calmly and quickly, first check respiration, pulse and treat for signs of shock (see page 188).

Safely muzzle kitty if no breathing difficulties are present as even the gentlest pet could bite when enduring great pain.

Flush gently with or immerse burned areas in cool (not ice) water while you are checking on the phone with your Veterinarian for further instructions. Burns can continue to cause damage even after the initial source of the burn has been removed. The flow of cool water reduces temperature below the skin surface to help prevent further damage, but it must be done slowly over a period of time rather than taking quick measures with ice which could lower your cat's body temperature or add frostbite to the injuries.

Pat dry with a soft cloth (not cotton balls which leave fibers behind).

Bandage loosely (or wrap in a clean sheet but use non-stick pad closest to burn if possible) to keep clean and prevent anything from entering damaged tissue and seek veterinary help immediately.

DO NOT apply any gels, ointments or sprays until seen by a Veterinarian.

If no infection occurs, healing can occur as quickly as 3 weeks.

Third Degree Burns

SIGNS & SYMPTOMS:
- Surface of the skin will appear charred, white or leathery and brown (An unpleasant visual, but think black like a charred burger you left on the grill too long; white like a boiled chicken breast. Your cat's tissue has in fact cooked!)
- Swelling under the skin or absence of skin.
- Third degree burns go through all the layers of skin and into the muscle underneath.
- Pain, although sometimes due to the destruction of nerve endings, is not immediately as painful as 2nd degree burns.

WHAT YOU MAY NEED:
- Muzzle
- Room Temperature Water
- Non-Stick Gauze
- Gauze Rolls
- Adhesive Tape
- Clean White Sheet or Other Smooth Fabric

WHAT TO DO:
Seek immediate veterinary care but call first!

Intravenous fluids, antibiotics and hospitalization may be needed.

Calmly and quickly, first check respiration, pulse and treat for signs of shock (see page 188).

Safely muzzle if no breathing difficulties are present as an animal in severe pain may bite.

Flush gently with or immerse burned areas in cool (not ice) water while you are checking on the phone with your Veterinarian for further instructions. Burns can continue to cause damage even after the initial source of the burn has been removed. The flow of cool water reduces temperature below the skin surface to help preventfurther damage but it must be done slowly over a period of time rather than taking quick measures with ice which could lower your cat's body temperature or add frostbite to the injuries.

Pat dry with a soft cloth (not cotton balls which leave fibers behind).

Bandage (or wrap in a clean sheet but use non-stick pad closest to burn if possible) to keep clean and prevent anything from entering damaged tissue and seek veterinary help immediately.

DO NOT apply any gels, ointments or sprays until seen by a Veterinarian.

During transport to the veterinary facility, monitor the animal for signs of shock (see page 188).

Chemical Burns

SIGNS & SYMPTOMS:
- Can exhibit signs of first, second or third degree burns (see previous pages) with the addition of a foreign substance (chemical) on the fur or skin.

WHAT YOU MAY NEED:
- Room Temperature Water
- Liquid Dish Soap or Shampoo
- Cold Pack
- Aloe Vera Gel or Triple Antibiotic Cream
- Non-Stick Gauze
- Gauze Rolls
- Adhesive Tape
- Clean White Sheet or Other Smooth Fabric
- Blunt-nosed Scissors
- Disposable Gloves for You
- Goggles or Eye Protection

WHAT TO DO:

Protect yourself first, if you are injured then you are no help to your cat. Put on disposable gloves and use protective eyewear in case the animal shakes or the chemical you are removing splashes into your eyes or on to your skin.

If available, read chemical label for appropriate treatment. Otherwise, flush liquid chemicals from pet's body with large amounts of room temperature water for at least 10 minutes (water that is too hot may speed up the absorption of the chemical through the skin while water that is too cold can cause hypothermia).

- If you believe that an animal in your care has been exposed to a chemical agent that may affect their lungs, seek veterinary care immediately.
- If chemical is oily/greasy, gently massage dishwashing liquid into the fur/skin first to dissolve grease before flushing with water. Take care as if the chemical has reached skin, your pet may be sore to the touch.
- If it is a dry chemical (powdered or granular), brush away or even vacuum out of the animal's fur if he will allow you to do so safely. Adding water may further activate the chemical so do not flush with water until any dry chemical has been removed. This even applies to laundry soap which is easier to remove in bulk while dry than when it lathers. Lathered soaps may also be strong and burn your pet's skin, so brush away first.
- Seek veterinary assistance immediately if the burn appears to be second or third degree (as described on page 140).
- Bring the chemical container (if possible) with you to the veterinary facility in a zip lock bag or by other safe method of transport.

Electrical Burns

CONDITION OVERVIEW:

A cat who receives an electric shock may have burns and/or the shock may cause an irregular heartbeat resulting in cardiac arrest. Damage may also occur to the capillaries in the lungs leading to fluid accumulation (pulmonary edema) causing respiratory difficulties or failure.

Do not touch an animal that is/has been electrocuted until the electricity (circuit breaker) is off or the source of electrocution (wires) has been safely moved away with a non-conducive material such as wood or plastic.

PREVENTIVE MEASURES/CAUSES:

- Place cords in locations inaccessible to pets or unplug when not in use
- Use outlet covers
- Cover cords with plastic sleeves or special tubing
- Teach cats NOT to chew and provide other appropriate chewing activities for teething kitties

- Unconscious
- Belabored breathing
- Visible burns or wounds
- Bite marks on an electrical cord or a burning odor in the room could imply your cat was burned or received a shock

WHAT YOU MAY NEED:
- Gauze Squares, Rolls & Adhesive Tape or Flexible Wrap
- Non-Conductive stick to move away electrical wires

WHAT TO DO:
Immediately check if the animal is breathing and has a pulse.

If the animal is not breathing, administer rescue breathing or CPCR (if heartbeat is also absent) and get to your Veterinarian immediately.

Even if the animal is conscious after electrocution, it is still advisable to seek veterinary attention because even minor electrical shocks can damage blood vessels in the lungs which could cause a slow leak of fluid that can make breathing difficult. It can take any where from several hours to a few days before symptoms (shortness of breath, loss of appetite, lethargy) set in. Do not delay veterinary care.

Check the animal for burns to the face or in the mouth, and provide wound treatment (See Bleeding Injuries page 122).

BUMPS & LUMPS

CONDITION OVERVIEW:
Lumps are often a concern – they are easy to feel and make cat parents think something is wrong with their furry child. Lumps are divided into two groups:

- Benign – Non-cancerous lumps may grow bigger but do not spread elsewhere.

- Malignant - Aggressive cancerous lumps which not only grow but also spread through the body and may affect vital organs.

The most common lumps are lipomas (benign fatty tumors), papillomas (wart-like growths or tags) and sebaceous cysts (which often drain a creamy fluid). Sometimes benign lumps are removed as they can be a nuisance if they continue to grow by restricting the movement of a leg or joint, pressing on the airway or other organs.

Mammary tumors can appear on both males and females and should be removed, but if found early, may not be problematic.

Mast cell tumors can be benign but are most often malignant and should generally be removed before they spread to other areas of the body.

PREVENTIVE MEASURES/CAUSES:

- Read labels on products used around your cat
- Dose flea repellants and other medications properly
- Perform weekly head-to-tail check-ups to find trouble spots early
- Don't skip annual veterinary visits
- Talk to your Veterinarian about titer tests before getting annual vaccinations
- Provide a nutritious diet with high quality protein, no fillers, food colorings or cancer causing preservatives

SIGNS & SYMPTOMS:

- Abnormal swellings that persist or continue to grow
- Sores that won't heal
- Weight loss
- Loss of appetite, difficulty eating or swallowing
- Bleeding or discharge from any opening on the body
- Offensive odor
- Reluctance to exercise or tires quickly
- Lameness or stiffness that won't go away
- Difficulty breathing, urinating or defecating

If you suspect anything is "not quite right" with your cat, it is best to have your medical professional check her out immediately.

WHAT YOU MAY NEED:

- Veterinary appointment

WHAT TO DO:

Follow veterinary instructions

Many things can cause a lump – bruising, swelling caused by fluid build-up, hematomas (blood filled sacs), abscesses (sacs of pus often near puncture wounds), ticks, foxtails or any protrusion. You can't tell just by looking at it even if you are a Veterinarian! However, there are several clues that may help your vet decide whether a lump on your pet is likely to be benign or malignant:

- If the lump moves (i.e., if it can be picked up in the fingers and moved around), it is less likely to be aggressive, ***but only your Veterinarian can tell for sure***.

- If the lump is firm, fast growing and does not move, it is more likely to be malignant as these lumps grow into the tissue below the skin, ***but only your Veterinarian can tell for sure***.

If the lump is red, painful when touched or is discharging fluid and if your pet seems to not be feeling well, get it checked out immediately. Testing a lump can be as easy as putting a needle into it to collect a few cells or your Veterinarian may feel it is necessary to take a piece of the lump under anesthesia to best determine what kind of lump it is. Once the type is known, your Veterinarian will be able to advise you on the best treatment for your pet.

One in every five cats will suffer from cancer with lymphoma, with lymphoma (associated with feline leukemia) being most common along with tumors and oral squamous carcinoma. When certain canine cancers are discovered early, the probability of a positive outcome can be good. Every year advances are made and feline cancer research, so do those head-to-tail check-ups weekly and don't miss an annual visit to your Veterinarian!

<u>Cancer Primer</u>

Hemangiosarcoma is most commonly found in the spleen, liver and heart. Prognosis is determined by location of the disease.

Adenocarcinomas present in the anal sacs on either side of the rectum. Size can range greatly and symptoms vary depending upon gender of the pet but can include increased thirst, weakness, persistent licking at the site, difficulty defecating and decreased appetite.

Lymphoma is cancer of the lymphatic tissue which is a core part of the body's immune system. The most common sign is a painless enlargement of the lymph nodes.

Mast cell tumors are among the most common tumors found in dogs generally found on the skin, spleen, liver and bone marrow but contain chemicals that can be released into surrounding tissue. They vary greatly in size, shape, appearance and texture. The only way to definitively identify is through a biopsy.

Osteosarcoma is the most common bone tumor in dogs, less so in cats, but can spread throughout the blood stream early on (metastasis). Frequently, it's found in the wrist, shoulder, knee and hip. Lameness due to pain followed by swelling are first signs.

Sarcomas Soft tissue sarcomas are a group of several different types of tumors made of connective tissue (bone, muscle, joint). They are located either within the skin, or in tissues just below the skin so are often discovered when petting or grooming your furry friend.

Squamous cell carcinoma occurs in the mouth, under the tongue and along the gum line in middle-aged and older cats. Common signs include difficulty eating, drooling and odor from the mouth.

Transitional cell carcinoma tumors usually form at the bladder opening causing painful urination. Cats often strain or may have blood in the urine making it difficult to diagnose since these are the same symptoms for urinary tract infections, which often delays diagnosis.

CLOTHES DRYER INJURIES

CONDITION OVERVIEW:
Burns, broken bones, abrasions, heat stroke, breathing/suffocation and cardiac arrest can occur when a cat curls up in a warm clothes dryer to sleep, and his unwary owner throws a load of clothes on top of her and starts the dryer.

PREVENTIVE MEASURES/CAUSES:
- Make it a habit to keep the washer and dryer closed when not in use, and always check inside before using. Follow the same practice with refrigerators and freezers. Cats are curious creatures and they can quickly jump into one of those appliances when your back is turned. Be diligent when you have a four-legged "toddler" and make sure his environment is safe.

SIGNS & SYMPTOMS:
- Burns/Singed fur
- Redness, pain, wounds/abrasions
- Broken bones
- Cardiac and/or pulmonary arrest

WHAT YOU MAY NEED:
- Teflon Coated Gauze Squares
- Gauze Rolls
- Water
- Splinting Materials (popsicle sticks, unsharpened pencils, wooden spoons, rolled up magazines, bubble wrap, to name just a few, in addition to an actual Sam Splint®)

WHAT TO DO:
Check if cat is conscious and breathing. If not, immediately administer CPR. If pet is alert, treat according to injuries (cool burns with water), splint or place on back board if you suspect broken bones and get to the Veterinarian immediately.

CONSTIPATION

CONDITION OVERVIEW:
Difficult or infrequent bowel movements are painful and hazardous to your cat. Healthy kitty cats have 1-2 stools per day so a day or two without is a cause for concern. When an animal is constipated, toxins remain in the body.

PREVENTIVE MEASURES/CAUSES:
- Pay attention to your cat and monitor bathroom habits. You won't know if your cat is relieving herself appropriately if you let her run stray in the neighborhood. Check litter boxes and and if you have multiple kitties, become acquainted with their habits so you know who is doing what.

- Do not give pets cooked bones, which not only can puncture but can also block the intestines.
- Monitor pets around toys and notice if articles of clothing are missing -- in other words, keep items that might tempt your pet out of paws reach.
- Make sure cats are provided a diet with some fiber and plenty of fresh water at all times.
- Minimize furballs by brushing kitty daily.

SIGNS & SYMPTOMS:
- Cat is straining to go with no results or crying in pain
- Hard stools, possibly covered with mucous or blood
- Lethargy
- Vomiting
- Abdominal discomfort
- Dehydration
- Enlarged colon
- Arthritis
- Hypothyroidism (thyroid deficiency)

WHAT YOU NEED:
- Sugar-Free Bran Cereal
- Canned Pumpkin Puree * (not pumpkin pie mix which has added sugars and ingredients)

*TIP: When opening a can of pumpkin, spoon left-overs into an ice cube tray and freeze. Then pop frozen 1 tablespoon servings into a zip lock bag and keep in the freezer until next time. Dehydrated varieties are also available so that you may mix up only as much as needed and some contain apple fiber which also aids in elimination.

WHAT TO DO:
If this is a first time occurrence, try one of the following methods of relief:
- Keep your cat well hydrated by encouraging water consumption.
- Feed 1 tablespoon sugar-free bran cereal for a cat; check with your Veterinarian but Metamucil®-type wafers are often a good choice.
- The authors' personal favorite home remedy is to feed pureed cooked pumpkin! Give 1 tablespoon to a cat. Most pets like the smooth texture and the fiber pushes things through the colon! If animal has not resumed normal bowel movements in 24 hours, seek veterinary care.

NOTE: Giving cats ½-1 teaspoon of cooked pure pumpkin daily also assists in the elimination of furballs along with good brushing.

COUGHING

CONDITION OVERVIEW:

Coughing is a reflex resulting from an irritation in the airway. People cough to eliminate dust, bacteria and itchy things from our throats and windpipes, but for cats coughing is unusual. While coughing up the occasional hairball isn't anything to worry about, coughing that lasts a day or more could be the sign of a respiratory infection, bronchitis, or congestive heart failure, so don't delay in getting your pet to the Veterinarian!

PREVENTIVE MEASURES/CAUSES:

- Adjust collars and leashes so that they don't restrict the trachea.
- Observe pets while they are eating and playing with toys to make sure they don't become choking obstructions.
- Take notice of chemical, fumes, and foods that might be irritating your pet.
- At the first sign of distress in your pet, have him checked out by his medical professional.

SIGNS & SYMPTOMS:

- Wet/moist cough could indicate fluid or phlegm in the lungs.
- Choking cough, with pawing at mouth could mean the pet is choking (page 129) or collar is too tight.
- Do not smoke in the presence of your pets as they can develop emphysema from second-hand smoke.
- Observe your pet's reaction to aerosol sprays, cleaners, fertilizers and chemicals of any type used around your house and yard. Many will irritate your pet resulting in coughing or breathing difficulties.
- Prolonged coughing at night or while lying down could suggest heart disease.

WHAT YOU MAY NEED:

- A calm demeanor to check throat for obstructions or loosen collar
- Humidifier
- Honey
- Lemon
- Water

WHAT TO DO:

Take collar off. An irritated airway will benefit from less pressure being placed on it. Instead use a harness to keep your cat safe if she must go outdoors with you..

If your kitty is experiencing a dry cough, humidify the air or sit with her in the bathroom while you run the shower to moisten up the room and his airway.

Administer a natural cough syrup! 1 teaspoon honey mixed with1 teaspoon of lemon in a ½ cup of water. Give it to your feline twice daily or more frequently if needed.

A wonderful herb that can prove helpful in eliminating coughing and fluid build-up is Dandelion. The leaves have a diuretic property, that removes excess fluid from the body. Find a quality health food store and give 2 drops per pound of your pet's body weight of the tincture twice daily.

If the cough lasts more than a day or two, take your pet to the Veterinarian as it could be serious or at least require additional meds. Don't purchase OTC cough syrups without veterinary advice as many contain acetaminophen, aspirin or other hidden ingredients. Two homeopathic remedies your Veterinarian may suggest are *Belladona* for a dry cough and *Pulsatilla* for a cough that is dry at night and loose (productive meaning fluid is being coughed up) in the morning.

CPCR (CARDIO PULMONARY CEREBRAL RESUSCITATION)

Please refer to page 105 in this handbook.

DEAFNESS

CONDITION OVERVIEW:
Are doorbells and electric can openers no longer getting a rise out of your cat? Do you find your pet is easily startled when you enter a room? For an animal to hear sounds, cells that transmit vibrations as well as the brains cells that interpret them, must be intact and functioning properly.

Birth defects, disease, injury and even medication can cause animals to lose hearing. A Veterinarian can assess and determine the correct course of action, but don't lose heart… pets are remarkably adaptable and can often hear something if you find the right pitch.

Fluffy may no longer hear those low mellow tones, but she might be able to discern a higher pitch if used to call her name.

PREVENTIVE MEASURES/CAUSES:
- Inspect your kitty's ears weekly or anytime she comes in from the outdoors.
- Place a large cotton ball in your cat's ears when bathing to avoid fluid build-up and fungal infections. Keep your pet's ears free of wax which can block the ear canals, but never use a cotton swab as you could damage the ear drum.
- Only use medications as prescribed.

SIGNS & SYMPTOMS:
- No longer obeys commands, seems to wander aimlessly or looks confused.
- White coat and/or blue eyes: About half of all white cats are deaf, and those numbers increase in cats with blue eyes, with deafness often found on the same side as the blue eye.

WHAT YOU MAY NEED:
- Your hands! Clap behind dog to see if there is a response.
- Whistle or other noise makers to test your pet's range of hearing.

WHAT TO DO:

Veterinary check-up where your pet professional can assess cause and degree of deafness and determine if any medical treatments are an option.

Help your precious kitty adjust to a new yet good quality life...

- Always walk your cat on a leash if she must go outside and keep her out of harm's way
- Teach her signals: "Come" by waving your hand towards yourself or flicking the kitchen light switch on and off for instance.
- Gently stomp your feet when you approach so as not to startle your pet. Owners sometimes believe their cat is getting cranky or aggressive she in fact she is just startled by someone she didn't hear coming. Approach deaf pets head-on, so that you are seen, and create vibrations so that they won't be caught off guard and nip to protect themselves.
- Get your four-legged friend a four-legged companion whose cues she can follow to know when someone is at the door.
- Most important of all, however, is to be patient with your best friend who is going through a transition and needs your continued love and support.

DEHYDRATION

CONDITION OVERVIEW:

Dehydration can be fatal as water is essential to all living beings! It makes up 3/4 of your pet's body and aids in circulation, digestion and the elimination of toxins. When your cat is over-heated from exercise or temperature, or when she is ill and suffering from vomiting or diarrhea, she can lose up to 10% of his body weight quickly through fluid loss. Elderly, pregnant or nursing cats and ones with diabetes are most prone to dehydration.

PREVENTIVE MEASURES/CAUSES:

- Hydrate, hydrate, hydrate! Always make sure your kitty has plenty of cool fresh water available and monitor her drinking habits...she should consume about 1 ounce of water for every pound she weighs daily! Make sure her water bowl is washed daily with warm soap and water and never goes dry. Daily put out fresh water in a mug or glass on a counter top your kitty frequents to encourage drinking. Many cats don't like bowls that touch their whiskers.
- Tune in to your cat so as to alert to increased body temperature, runny stools or even constipation (which could imply inadequate fluid intake).
- Endocrine diseases such as Addison's and diabetes can contribute.

SIGNS & SYMPTOMS:

- Gums feel dry or sticky to the touch.
- Tugor Test -- Skin stays in a "tent" or falls back in place slowly rather than snapping back when you gently pull up on it over your pet's neck and upper back.
- Sunken eyes
- Lethargy
- Loss of appetite
- Depression
- Delayed Capillary Refill Time

WHAT YOU MAY NEED:
- Needle-less Syringe, Eye Dropper or even clean spray bottle with water
- Electrolyte Solution (pet brands exist or make your own below)
    - 1 Quart Fresh Water (bottled or filtered preferred)
    - 1 Tablespoon Honey
    - 1 Teaspoon Salt

Mix and store in refrigerator but serve at room temperature making a fresh batch daily. Throughout the day, dose:

- 3 Tablespoons for kittens
- 5 Tablespoons for pets up to 5 lbs.
- 3/4 cups for pets up to 10 lbs.
- 1/4 cup per 5 lbs. of body weight for pets 15 lbs. and more

To keep on hand, mix 4 cups water with 1 teaspoon salt and 1 teaspoon sugar and freeze in ice cube trays.

WHAT TO DO:
If cat's temperature is normal (100.4°F – 102.5° F) encourage her to drink or offer her some electrolyte solution. If temperature is higher, dribble small amounts of solution through a syringe onto tongue or spray small amount of water into mouth. Dehydration can be very serious!

DIABETES

CONDITION OVERVIEW:
Is your kitty thirstier than usual or eating more? Is she running to the litter box more frequently or not making it there in time? Cats produce a hormone called insulin that enables their cells to secrete glucose which is used as fuel. Animals with diabetes either don't produce enough insulin or the insulin they do make doesn't work efficiently meaning their cells do not get the fuel they need. Obesity, pancreatitis, hyperthyroidism and poisons can contribute to this condition. Also see Blood Sugar Issues on page 137.

PREVENTIVE MEASURES/CAUSES:
- Get annual check-ups at your Veterinarian and at the sign of increased thirst or urination.
- Don't overfeed sugary items to your cat.

SIGNS & SYMPTOMS:
- Increased thirst and urination
- Unusually sweet breath

In later stages:
- Loss of appetite
- Vomiting
- Lethargy and Coma
- Rare muscle weakness in cats where they walk down on their hocks rather than up on their toes

WHAT YOU MAY NEED:
- Insulin as prescribed.
- Honey or Karo® Syrup
- Appropriate diet

WHAT TO DO:

Have your Veterinarian confirm diabetes through blood and urine testing.

Follow prescribed regime of insulin injections or other medications. Stay on schedule!

Keep your pet at a healthy weight and well exercised.

Feed smaller meals more frequently to keep blood sugar at an even keel and switch to a high-fiber diet if recommended by your pet's health care provider.

Giving insulin can sometimes cause blood sugar to plummet (hypoglycemia) so with a diabetic cat, always have honey or Karo® Syrup on hand to rub on your pet's gums should he suddenly get shaky. (See LOW BLOOD SUGAR page 137).

DIARRHEA & VOMITING

CONDITION OVERVIEW:

Although vomiting and diarrhea are both common signs of many poisons and illnesses, most often they are caused by simple digestive upsets -- your pet ate too much, too fast or something that was spoiled like out of the garbage can. Items ranging from moldy bread to rotten apples can upset your pet's stomach. Frequent loose or liquid bowel movements can come on quickly and last only a brief period of time. Ongoing bouts of diarrhea, however, can lead to dehydration and may indicate an underlying health concern. Pay attention to your pet's bodily habits. Check your cat's litter box daily for activity to stay on top of their health and well-being.

Knowing the difference between vomiting and regurgitation can help your Veterinarian evaluate what is up with your pussy cat. Vomiting occurs when food or liquid, is expelled from your pet's stomach or upper small intestine and is generally preceded by audible retching. If it originated in the stomach, it may include clear liquid while yellow or green liquid clues you in that it came from the small intestine. Of course undigested or partially digested food may also come forth.

Regurgitation differs in that the expelled material almost always comes from the esophagus (the muscular tube that propels water, food and saliva downward into the stomach). When your pet regurgitates, he brings up water, saliva and undigested food silently and the suddenness of it takes you both by surprise. A concern though is that since it occurs quickly, the larynx (opening to the windpipe) often doesn't have time to close and some of the regurgitated matter can be inhaled into the lungs resulting in aspiration pneumonia.

PREVENTIVE MEASURES/CAUSES:

- Regularly get down on all fours and check your house and yard , as well as look up on counter tops and shelves, for items your cat might get into or even absorb through his paws, and do your doggone best to keep dangers out of paws reach!
- Prevent your cat from drinking water from lakes, streams, out of gutters, buckets and unsanitary sources. Wash her water bowl with warm water and soap daily.
- Don't feed table scraps (fat, grease, salts or rich foods) or change your cat's diet suddenly.
- Reduce stress in your cat's life as well as in your own.
- Provide regular check-ups making sure titers are high (see page 46) or vaccines are up-to-date so that your pets won't contract disease.

SIGNS & SYMPTOMS:

- Loose or frequent stools sometimes containing blood mucus
- Flatulence
- Straining or urgency to go
- Weight loss
- Dehydration
- Fever
- Lethargy
- Vomiting

WHAT YOU MAY NEED:

- Antacid
- Syringe or tablespoon to measure
- Electrolytes
- Plenty of fresh water
- Pumpkin Puree * (not pumpkin pie mix which has added sugars and ingredients)
- Ginger Snap Cookies, Ginger Root or Capsules

WHAT TO DO:

If an animal in your care is experiencing vomiting and/or diarrhea and you know that it is not the result of poisoning:

- Rest the stomach by withholding food for 24 hours but always provide fresh water to prevent dehydration. Pedialyte® (diluted 50/50 with water) or a pet-specific electrolyte replenisher (see recipe for homemade version on page 151) can replace minerals taken out of the body due to diarrhea or vomiting.
- Administer antacid every 4-6 hours…For cats, the best bet is to get a prescription from your veterinarian.

- Pumpkin puree is a beneficial natural cure as most animals like the taste and the fiber helps firm up loose stools. Dose 1 tablespoon for small dogs and cats and up to 3 tablespoons for a large dog.
- Ginger! Ginger snap cookies (human kind are usually the easiest to dose and can also cure an upset tummy.) Half a cookie generally does the trick. As for pure ginger capsules…50 mg for every 10 lbs. your cat weighs repeated every 6-8 hours, or if Fluffy will drink, peel fresh ginger root, make 5-8 ¼" thick slices and boil in ¼ cup water. When it cools, let him lap it up. Any of these ginger tips may also work if administered 20-30 minutes before a road trip to keep motion sickness at bay.
- If all is well in 24 hours, you probably have a hungry animal on your hands so feed a bland diet for a few days (plain steamed rice and boiled white chicken is a good option) before getting pet back on his regular diet.
- If vomiting/diarrhea persist beyond 24 hours, or if at any time you notice blood, get to your Veterinarian and bring a vomit/diarrhea sample along.

HOMEOPATHIC TIPS: For gastrointestinal distress or even pancreatitis, along with veterinary care, *Nux Vomica* (commonly known as Strychnine Tree) given 2x daily can help. For diarrhea, *Arsenicum Album* (1 30c tablet per 20 lbs. of body weight every 4 hours) is a good choice or Phosphorous if there is blood in the stool such as with colitis. Incorporating western herbs such as *Slippery Elm* can aid with Irritable Bowel Syndrome, Diarrhea and Constipation while aloe vera is beneficial for gas and acid reflux – dried form is better tolerated by animals than the gel. Additionally, chamomile or peppermint can be made into a tea to settle tummies and rehydrate. Give 1 tablespoon for every 10 lbs. your pet weighs repeating every 4-6 hours.

DROWNING

CONDITION OVERVIEW:

Drowning occurs when there is an accumulation of fluid in the lungs, typically when an animal is immersed in a body of water but it can also occur on dry land when fluid is aspirated into the lungs. With water in the lungs, there is no room for oxygen and suffocation occurs. Submersion time, water temperature as well as whether it was fresh, salt or chemical water will affect the prognosis. Some pets recover from near drowning incidents only to develop fluid in the lungs (pulmonary edema) hours later. Known as "dry drowning," this too can be fatal so anytime your pet has fallen into water, have him checked out by your veterinary professional at once!

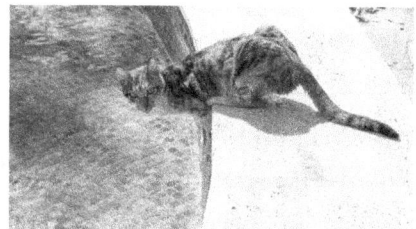

PREVENTIVE MEASURES/CAUSES:

- Not all cats know how to swim – it's not an innate trait! Make any water environment safe for Fluffy by fencing it off, attaching a pet ramp to the side of swimming pools or making pets wear a life-jacket when at the lake or boating. Even good swimmers tire, and since they can't rest with paws on the bottom nor tread water, a jacket can help keep them afloat.

- Refresh those pets that swim each season as to where the way out of the pool is! Yes, some cats are aquatic athletes and enjoy it, believe it or not?!
- Keep your eyes on your pets at all times when they are near the water. Accidents only take seconds to occur. Your cat could fall through ice, get caught in a flood, suffer a head injury or seizure while in or near the water.
- Never force water into an animal trying to make her drink. Administer slowly with a needle-less syringe or eye dropper when trying to hydrate so as not to aspirate fluid into the lungs..

SIGNS & SYMPTOMS:
- If you find an animal in a body of water, get them out!
- Blue gums/skins
- Coughing with clear to red foam
- Crackling sound from the chest
- Unconscious to barely conscious
- Difficulty breathing or absence of breathing and pulse

WHAT YOU MAY NEED:
- Towel, rope, life preserver, Skimmer pole with a net -- something to help you get the cat out of the water but if he is conscious and struggling, take appropriate measures so that they do not pull you under
- Cushions, folded towels to elevate hind quarters on larger animals
- Towels, blankets to warm pet in
- Karo Syrup® or Honey
- Calm demeanor to perform necessary tasks to help your best friend
- Transportation to veterinary help

WHAT TO DO:
Quickly remove animal from water. If kitty is struggling, it is best for you not to enter but rather stay near shore or pool side so that she won't pull you under in her state of panic.

Hold cats securely by the hind legs to drain water from lungs, windpipe and mouth. Next lay kitty on her side and elevate…with folded towel to help drain water.

If you detect a heartbeat but the animal is not breathing, begin rescue breathing immediately. Wrap the animal in towels or blankets to keep from going into hypothermia and continue rescue breathing until the cat shows signs of recovery or until a veterinary professional can take over. Oddly enough, research has shown that water 90° F and below can slow the rate at which brain cells die, so some animals that have spent a considerable time in cold water have a good chance at recovery.

If the animal is not breathing and there is an absent heartbeat, begin CPCR and get prompt veterinary attention. Do not stop CPCR unless the animal shows signs of recovery or until a veterinary professional can take over. If you have additional hands, rub Karo ® Syrup or honey on the pet's gums which could aid in resuscitation.

Even when you are lucky enough to revive Fluffy, immediately follow-up with a veterinary visit for assessment of any life-threatening inflammation to the lungs.

EMBEDDED OBJECTS

CONDITION OVERVIEW:
Due to their inquisitive nature and scavenging habits, our pets are likely to get a foreign object embedded in their skin. Glass, thorns, needles and sticks are most common, but could include an arrow or quill from a porcupine. Removing an object that is penetrating deeply could result in massive blood loss and tissue damage, so first aid may include securing it in place and acquiring immediate medical attention.

PREVENTIVE MEASURES/CAUSES:
- Keep your yard clear of dangers and watch your cat's area for shining glass, bramble or anything that could puncture paws or any body part.
- Monitor cats around lakes where there could be fishhooks or other sharp objects.
- Take special care in places like garages and workshops where many small but sharp items can be easily dropped.
- Don't allow pets near locations where bow & arrow shooting may occur.

WHAT YOU MAY NEED:
- Gauze squares & rolls
- Adhesive tape or flexible wrap
- Tweezers
- Paper or Styrofoam cup; empty margarine tub
- Disposable gloves
- Scissors
- Saline solution or purified water to clean
- Triple anti-biotic cream
- Towel or board to carry injured animal to transportation

WHAT TO DO:
If you find an animal in the unfortunate situation of having a stick, arrow or other object embedded in a body part:
- Keep the cat as still as possible. Remember that like many other times first aid is in order, you may need to restrain and muzzle the animal (see page 98).
- If it is a small object and doesn't appear to be too deeply embedded, remove with tweezers, clean and bandage (see page 122).
- If object is large or deep in skin and area is bleeding externally, secure the object in the exact position it is in by placing gauze rolls on each side and wrapping with a third roll.
- Make this wrap snug enough to hold the object in place but not tight enough to restrict blood flow or breathing. The idea is to secure the object so that it won't move and cause further tissue damage while you are transporting the cat to the Veterinarian. You can also make a ring bandage by first tying a triangular bandage into a tiny loop, and then wrapping each of the "tails" around the loop to form a ring. Finally tying those ends together and placing ring around embedded object to keep it in place.
- An alternative would be to brace the embedded object in place by cutting a hole in the top or slit the side of a plastic margarine tub or Styrofoam cup – the slit allows the object to penetrate up and through the container but remain still. Then tape the container firmly to the pet's body to prevent movement as removing objects sometimes cause great loss of blood so it is best done under professional medical care.

- Do not attempt to brace or stabilize an imbedded object if the cat is struggling, resistant or showing obvious signs of extreme pain and/or aggression. The animal could either cause the object to become imbedded further or cause physical harm to you (the first-responder).
- Transport the animal to the veterinary hospital immediately.

EYE INJURIES

CONDITION OVERVIEW:
A variety of eye issues can befall our four-legged friends: scratches to the cornea, cherry eye (oval pink mass of flesh protruding from the eye), entropion (portion of the eyelid is inverted or folded inward irritating the cornea), prolapse (eye comes out of socket) or blood-filled eye due to rupture of capillaries (subjunctive hematoma). With the exception of a speck of dirt or debris which can be flushed away, these injuries are best dealt with at your Veterinarian's office. As our cats age (and sometimes earlier) cloudiness or hardening of the cornea develops. Once again, your veterinary professional is key to helping your pet maintain sufficient vision and comfort.

PREVENTIVE MEASURES/CAUSES:
- Take note of toys your cat plays with – stiff nylon whiskers and other sharp parts should be cut off of stuffed animals so as not to scratch her eye when she plays with them.
- Observe your cat anytime she rubs her eye on the ground or with his paw. Tiny claws from other animals may scratch (raccoons are the most vicious). Running through hedges which are nothing but small sticks and possible sharp leaves can also cause damage to delicate corneal tissue. Catch problems early and have your Veterinarian care for it in a timely manner.
- Upper respiratory infections and other illnesses can cause redness, swelling and even prolapse so know your pet to quickly identify anything that is not quite right.

SIGNS & SYMPTOMS:
- Redness, pawing at the eye, rapid blinking, swelling
- Excessive tearing or any discharge
- Clouded cornea (the front clear covering of the eye)
- Unequally dilated pupils or lack of response of pupils could be a medical emergency

WHAT YOU MAY NEED:
- Eye Wash (Saline or Purified Water)
- Gauze squares
- Non-stick Gauze if covering eye
- Adhesive tape or flexible wrap

WHAT TO DO:

Cleanse the eye with sterile eye wash by pulling upwards on top lid to open eye wide and flushing from outer corner of eye making sure extra fluid and debris run down muzzle. Let kitty blink out extra liquid. Inspect in good light to make sure the foreign object has been removed.

If the eye is out of the socket or blood is present, cover with non-stick gauze dampened with eye wash and get to professional help immediately.

Do not attempt to pull ANYTHING that is penetrating eye ball. If it does not flush away, bandage in place (without applying additional pressure) and get quickly to your Veterinarian!

FALLS & HIGH RISE SYNDROME

CONDITION OVERVIEW:

Contrary to popular belief, cats do not always land on their feet. Many are injured from falls, so take care to prevent the worst from happening to your feline friend. From a fall out a window, off of a balcony or from a rooftop, cats can sustain a variety of injuries including broken bones, jaws, ruptured organs and even death. If you notice your cat is limping or refusing to move or eat, it is possible that she could have suffered an internal injury that may not be easily noticed but can become dangerous very quickly.

Our feline friends have a fluid-filled organ in their inner ear called the vestibular apparatus that helps them "right" themselves during a fall. When they topple from heights, cats sometimes "parachute" loose folds of skin under their legs relaxing those parts so that the abdomen and chest absorb more of the impact rather than their head and legs. When cats fall shorter distances most tend to land on their feet with legs rigid, resulting in multiple fractures, chest, jaw and spinal injuries, concussions and even ruptures of the internal organs. Either way, it is not a good thing for your furry friend and can prove life-threatening.

Dogs are even more likely to be injured in the event of a fall. Their bodies are denser than cat's and they do not generally right themselves which means they fall faster and harder, exponentially increasing the likelihood of severe injury.

PREVENTIVE MEASURES/CAUSES:

- Make sure you have screens securely in place on all windows and don't give pets unsupervised access to balconies, rooftops or other high places.
- Cats are climbers. Even if you don't live in "earthquake country," secure shelves, bookcases, television sets and anything that your feline friend might climb upon so that it can't fall when kitty jumps up.
- Don't place pets in harm's way for photo ops or other reasons. Four on the floor on sturdy ground is best!

SIGNS & SYMPTOMS:

Head Injuries:
- Confused/unstable
- Blood or clear cerebral spinal fluid coming out of ears, nose and/or eyes
- One pupil larger or pupils non-reactive to light

Spinal Injuries:
- Unstable, crooked stance of head/neck or paralysis
- Breathing & bleeding concerns

WHAT YOU MAY NEED:
- Gauze squares and gauze rolls
- Adhesive tape or flexible wrap
- Towel, board, cookie sheet (and strips of fabric to restrain animal to board) to move or lift pet
- Muzzle

WHAT TO DO:

Check to see if your cat is breathing. If not, administer rescue breathing by giving two quick breaths into his nose while closing his mouth. Make sure the chest rises. Then give breaths according to chart on page 105 until pet breathes on his own or you reach medical help.

Every 30 seconds, check for a pulse at her inner thigh (femoral artery) or by cupping your hand behind the front elbow at the chest feeling for heart beat. If there is none, begin CPCR (see pages 105). Do realize though, this is not a cure, and you must quickly get your cat to the Veterinarian even if she starts breathing on her own. Transport her gently on a cutting board, cookie sheet or similar stiff object and secure her with rolled gauze so that she does not shift off of it.

If your pet is breathing, check for bleeding injuries. Apply direct pressure with a sterile gauze pad to stop external bleeding and prevent infection. If you notice a "sucking" chest wound (you'll see bubbling and hear air rushing into the body as your cat strains to breathe), wrap the body with plastic wrap to seal it and get your pet to the Veterinarian immediately -- do not delay. See Bleeding Injuries, Rescue Breathing, CPCR and Transporting an Injured Animal sections of this book for further details.

Realize any blood coming from or pooling in the eyes, nose or mouth could mean a head injury or internal bleeding requiring quick medical attention. Don't forget that a conscious animal in pain may bite even his most loyal human friend, so restrain his head with a towel or use a muzzle as long as it doesn't interfere with injuries.

FROSTBITE

CONDITION OVERVIEW:

Animals don't tell us when their paws get numb. We find out only when it hurts for them to step or when we notice tissue has become hard and dark. Frostbite is a condition that can occur as a result of exposure to freezing or subfreezing temperatures. It most commonly affects the tips of the ears, the tail, the scrotum and the paws, especially the toes. When your four-legged best friend is in a cold environment, their body responds by reducing blood flow to the extreme parts of their body. This provides good blood flow to their vital organs but decreases the oxygen and warmth in the extremities allowing ice crystals to form in the tissue.

PREVENTIVE MEASURES/CAUSES:

- Use common sense and limit time outdoors. When out with your cat, periodically warm ear flaps between your hands, check paws to keep snow and ice from between the toes and never let your faithful friend out in the winter without accompanying her.
- Short furred pets without under coats can benefit from a cat sweater when outside for even short periods of time.
- A temperature of 10° F or below is too cold for a cat to withstand, but there are just too many variables to predict at what temperature tissue damage will occur.
- Watch for hard tissue varying in color from pale to gray as this could mean frostbite and may not be detected unless the fur has sloughed off. Once the area defrosts, the skin will redden and become tender. In severe cases, the tissue turns black within a few days and dies.

WHAT YOU MAY NEED:

- Towels, blanket
- Clothes dryer
- Warm liquids and syringe to administer if they won't lap it up

WHAT TO DO:

Wrap frozen paws with blankets (tumbled briefly in a warm — not hot — clothes dryer) but do not massage area if tissue is hard as it will hurt. Never use a heating pad or hot water bottle as you may damage nerves and blood vessels.

Lower effected area (legs, paw, tail) by having pet lie in your lap or on a sofa to promote circulation to frostbitten parts.

Seek veterinary assistance immediately. As the tissue warms, frostbite turns painful, and Veterinarian Brooks Bloomfield of Truckee-Tahoe sadly explains, "Many of the pets I've seen had accelerated heart rates due to pain and some self-mutilated their paws and tail as the circulation returned." Therefore veterinary care is imperative. Additionally, antibiotics may be prescribed to prevent infection along with pain relief medication. In severe cases, amputation or surgical removal of affected tissue is not uncommon, so do all you can to keep your pet from becoming an icicle and help him live a longer, happier, healthier life with you!

HEAD ENTRAPMENT

CONDITION OVERVIEW:
Fido chases Fluffy or Fluffy dashes through a fence or gate only to find out that what went through will not come back out!

PREVENTIVE MEASURES/CAUSES:
- Examine your house and yard for fences, spaces between walls, pool equipment, work benches and any place your pet can get stuck or a body part trapped. Pets can outsmart us, but the more you pay attention to your environment from your pet's point of view, the more likely you are to see a possible accident waiting to happen.

SIGNS & SYMPTOMS:
- Head is stuck in a gate or fence and animal cannot move.

WHAT YOU MAY NEED:
- Patience and calming vibes to share with your pet
- Petroleum or K-Y® Jelly, baby oil or any type of grease to help slip your cat's head back through the barrier

WHAT TO DO:
Call your Animal Ambulance Service if needed, but first and foremost…stay calm and keep your pet calm as well. Rapid movements and jerking about can cause great damage to his head and neck. Kneel close to your cat, preferably positioning yourself behind her and holding her body close to what she is trapped in so as not to strain her neck by pulling on it. If she isn't having trouble breathing, muzzling might be a good idea to protect yourself.

Once she's relaxed, use a lubricant like K-Y or petroleum jelly to grease the fur of her neck and especially the crest of her skull (the thickest part of the head) as well as the bars/fencing that she is stuck in (even baby oil will work). This will help her slide and keep the fence rail or other object from scraping skin as the cat's head comes free.

If that isn't working and the bars or obstacle can be pried apart without causing pressure to the animal's head or neck, that would be an appropriate Plan B.

Provide follow-up care to any cuts or scrapes and if you fear there has been any neck or spinal injury, do not hesitate…get to your Veterinarian for x-rays.

When all is well, come up with a solution so that your cat can not become entrapped again.

HEAD PRESSING

CONDITION OVERVIEW:
The compulsive act of a cat pressing his head against a solid surface for extended periods of time. It generally indicates a nervous system problem or neurological illness or condition and should be evaluated by your Veterinarian at once.

PREVENTIVE MEASURES/CAUSES:
- Head Trauma
- Tumors or damage to the brain or skull including encephalitis
- Stroke
- Metabolic Disorder (Hyper or Hyponatremia – too much or too little sodium in the body's blood plasma)
- Toxic Poisoning
- Liver Disease
- Infection of the Nervous System (Rabies, Parasites, Bacterial, Fungal or Viral)

SIGNS & SYMPTOMS:
- Standing or lying with forehead pressed against a wall, sofa or other solid surface or pushing head into the ground
- Pacing or walking in circles
- Getting stuck in corners
- Staring at walls
- Visual problems
- Seizures
- Reflexes not functioning appropriately

WHAT YOU MAY NEED:
- Safe transport to the Veterinarian for diagnosis.

WHAT TO DO:
By recognizing the signs and getting an immediate veterinary evaluation, you just might save your pet's life.

HEAD SHAKING

CONDITION OVERVIEW:
When it comes to pets, any itch, sting or irritation may prompt them to shake their head in hopes of getting rid of the problem. An examination by you may determine the culprit, but a Veterinarian may be your only option for relief if the condition persists or seems debilitating.

PREVENTIVE MEASURES/CAUSES:
- Take care when cleaning ears that you don't squirt too much ear wash in that can't safely removed by you.
- When bathing cats, insert large cotton balls to prevent water from entering the canal.
- Perform weekly exams of the ears so as to catch an infection early.

SIGNS & SYMPTOMS:
- Continuous head shaking, scratching or pawing at the ear
- Head tilt

WHAT YOU MAY NEED:
- Flashlight
- Ear wash
- Soft cloth or gauze

WHAT TO DO:
Take a good look inside. Upon inspection you may notice the ear looks dirty OR red and infected OR smells bad OR you may find tiny black specks that could be the dirt from ear mites. If it seems dirty or there is wax build-up, give it a thoroughly cleaning as described in the Head-to-Tail exam portion of this book on page 118 by pouring ear wash onto a soft cloth and cleaning no deeper than the first knuckle on your index finger – no cotton swabs and take care not to push infection or debris into ear canal. If that doesn't do the trick, get to your Veterinarian for assistance. Middle ear infections can invade facial nerves and lead to facial paralysis; chronic infections can result in hearing loss and balance issues as well as meningitis, so don't delay in getting professional medical help.

If your cat has been outside there could also be foxtails or burrs trapped deep in the canal that only your Veterinarian can safely reach.

A head tilt may indicate a neurological problem, ear infection, irritation or be due to a toxin. Look inside your cat's ear and perform the tracking test learned on page 95, but most likely the best step is for your four-legged patient to receive medical care.

HEAT STROKE

CONDITION OVERVIEW:

Cats are more tolerant of heat than dogs, but it only takes a short period of time for an animal left in a car to get into a deadly situation. Pets don't sweat to regulate their body temperature (normally 100.0°F – 102.5°F). They release heat through their tongue, nose and foot pads. If a cat is panting, she is truly over-heated, in pain or possibly suffering from lung or heart disease, so the situation is serious! Pets pant to exchange cooler outside air with the warm humid air in their lungs while cats don't usually pant until they are overwhelmed by the heat. If the outside air isn't cooler than an animal's body temperature, the animal can succumb to heat stroke. Without prompt attention, heat stroke can result in brain damage, kidney failure, cardiac arrest and death.

PREVENTIVE MEASURES/CAUSES:

- Keep cats indoors in a temperate environment or on a shaded screened porch with cool air flow.
- NEVER leave your cat in a parked car for even a moment. If she can't get out with you at every stop, she is better off home in a temperate environment.
- Remember heating systems in winter can make kitty too hot.
- Get to know your groomer! Blow drying animals in a well-ventilated area is important to their health, and cage dryers (big boxes animals lie in with air forced in to dry them) must be carefully monitored, so choose a groomer you know has your pet's best interest at heart.
- Pay particular attention to senior, over-weight and brachycephalic (flat-faced Persians for instance) cats who have more difficulty breathing even at comfortable temperatures.

SIGNS & SYMPTOMS:

- Heavy panting
- Gasping
- Vomiting (if not yet dehydrated)
- Foam around the mouth
- Weak or high pulse
- Inability to drink
- Bright red or suddenly bluish gums
- Loss of consciousness

Heat stroke is a life-threatening emergency that requires veterinary treatment. The goal is to remove the kitty from the source of the heat, prevent internal body temperature from continuing to rise and transporting to a Veterinarian as quickly as possible.

WHAT YOU MAY NEED:

- Water from a sink with running water
- Thermometer and lubricating gel
- Karo Syrup® or Honey

WHAT TO DO:

Move the animal to a cooler environment. Indoors is best with a cool fan blowing on your pet but even a shady sidewalk or grassy area can help.

Wet the cat with luke-warm water (not ice to avoid additional shock - see page 188). Think "From the paws up!" getting the paws, pits, groin and belly skin cooled first is most effective in bringing down the animal's body temperature. Water often skids off fur on breeds with undercoats and does not cool skin when applied to their back.

If you place your cat into a tub or pool, do not let the water rise higher than the belly. Immersing her to the neck will cause her to cool too quickly resulting in hypothermia.

Rubbing alcohol or witch hazel wiped onto the inner flaps of the ears and pads of the feet has an amazing cooling effect. Do not however douse with an entire bottle of rubbing alcohol which could cause a sudden change in body temperature and result in shock. Also avoid getting in any cuts or scrapes as both sting.

Placing a cool pack (or bag of frozen peas) on the cat's neck and groin can prove helpful in cooling him off as the cooled blood flowing to major arteries cools the rest of the body. Remove pack every few minutes to make sure you don't cause frost bite to animal's tissue.

Do not force pet to drink as she could aspirate fluid into her lungs. Dribble a little water from an eye dropper or spray bottle to keep her hydrated. At the Veterinarian's office, fluids will likely be administered subcutaneously (under the skin or intravenously).

Check your pet's temperature and if it is 104°F or higher, get to the Veterinarian immediately! Wrap the cat in a wet sheet or towel, place in her carrier and turn on car air conditioning and drive quickly but safely.

Should the cat go unconscious, rub a little honey or Karo Syrup® on her gums to increase blood sugar level, and be prepared to administer CPCR.

If the cat cools too quickly and temperature drops to 100°F, cover her with a blanket and place a 2-liter bottle filled with warm (not hot) water next to her as you transport her to the Animal ER.

HOMEOPATHIC TIP: *Belladonna*, a fever reducer also known as Night Shade, can prove beneficial in bringing temperature down but not as quickly as water and proper environment.

HOT SPOTS & LICK SORES

Cats seldom get hot spots, but they can develop red, wet sores that make their skin look raw. They can be caused by a wide range of things but are made worse by their licking and chewing at the spot. Bacteria grows and spreads quickly creating a wound that can be painful and problematic to heal.

PREVENTIVE MEASURES/CAUSES:
- Does your pet have OCLD? Stop Obsessive Compulsive Licking Disorder in its tracks!
- Parasite prevention is key as the itchiness caused by fleas and ticks leads to your pets chewing himself raw.

HOMEPATHIC TIP: Neem seed oil and human grade diatomaceous earth can keep fleas away from your pets. Insect-borne diseases can be a serious health risk to people and pets but there is controversy over the safety of applying commercial insecticides so these can be effective alternatives.

SIGNS & SYMPTOMS:
- Obsessive licking, chewing, scratching
- Red, sore skin that is not healing and may have an aroma

WHAT YOU MAY NEED:
- Scissors
- Gauze squares
- Green tea bag
- Warm water
- Antibacterial spray or cream
- Apple cider vinegar

WHAT TO DO:
Trim fur around sore with blunt-nosed scissors so that you can easily clean area with warm water. Gently pat the area dry with a soft cloth. Do not apply ointments to a hot spot as these products seal in infection while medications containing alcohol will burn in an open wound. Instead use an antibacterial spray or cream that dries up the sore or apply a tea bag (green tea, not herbal, that has cooled after being soaked for 5 minutes in hot water). The tannic acid is a natural astringent that dries and heals. Use this treatment 3-5 times per day until healed.

Another remedy includes applying apple cider vinegar directly to the hot spot 4 times daily. Soak it in a cloth and wipe the clipped area gently. The vinegar has anti-inflammatory as well as antibacterial properties.

When dry, bandage loosely or use a cone collar-like device to prevent pet from licking the area.

Hot spots that persist without obvious signs of improvement for more than 7 days should be evaluated by a Veterinarian.

IN HEAT (refer to "Birthing" section page 119 if you are past this stage)

CONDITION OVERVIEW:

Estrus, or "heat" is the stage in a cat's reproductive cycle during which she becomes receptive to mating. Her estrogen levels first increase and then sharply decrease, and mature eggs are released from the ovaries. The first "heat" usually occurs between 6 and 24 months of age and then occurs every 3 weeks in cats during "Kitten Season" – the warmer parts of the year (April – September, longer in some areas). Each cycle lasts between 6-10 days, however, the female is only receptive to the male during the last half of this period. The male, however, may be interested the whole time.

PREVENTIVE MEASURES/CAUSES:

- Unless you are a responsible breeder willing to find forever homes for all the animals born, spay your female (and neuter your males) before her first heat cycle to avoid possible health complications as well as to prevent the birth of more animals when so many already need homes.
- While "in heat," keep your female inaccessible to males realizing that if there is a male in the neighborhood, he will perform due diligence to get to your female.
- If you allow your pet to become pregnant, it is your responsibility to see her and her kittens through it comfortably and with all medical care necessary.

SIGNS & SYMPTOMS:

- During estrus your female my act nervous, be easily distracted or even more alert than usual. She may feel the need to urinate more frequently and will exhibit changes in her behavior caused by the shift in hormones.
- Blood-tinged discharge may come from the vagina and the vulva will appear swollen.
- Discharge will decrease and lighten in color when she is ready to initiate sexual interactions with her suitors.
- Female may offer her hind-quarters towards approaching males.

WHAT YOU MAY NEED:

- Disinfectant and paper towels to clean up floors from any discharge
- Kitty diapers may help keep floors and carpets clean
- Good containment to keep male cats away
- A calm & knowledgeable demeanor as well as other helping hands

WHAT TO DO:

Prevention is the key – spay your cat, but your most important task is to keep your female indoors and safe from escapes where she could be lost, injured or hit by a car while in search of a "boyfriend."

Offer diversions but spend time with your Miss. Keep doors and windows and fences secured.

Keep your female friend clean and mask the smell -- Chlorophyll tablets may help mask the odor of her cycle and keep Romeos away.

If cats have mated, NEVER attempt to separate them. After the act, it is common for animals to remain "connected" back-to-back for up to 30 minutes. You may endanger the felines and/or be bitten if you interfere once nature has taken its course, so just allow them to remain safe and do not interfere until they separate on their own.

MANGE

CONDITION OVERVIEW:

Mange is an inflammatory condition caused by the Demodex Mite (various types so tiny you cannot seem them with the naked eye). Mange can cause a small, red, hairless area or almost complete hair loss (alopecia) with big pimples and thickened oozing skin. It can sometimes even disrupt the immune system. Mange occurs when mites burrow under the hair follicles and skin. Demodectic mange is much more common in dogs than in cats and typically causes hair loss and scaling around the eyelids, corners of the mouth and front legs. A second form called Canine Sarcoptic Mange or Scabies occurs when pets are exposed to an infected animal. This type of mange is very contagious (to humans and animals) and very itchy. Only your Veterinarian can tell you for sure which type of mange your pet has, so see him right away and be patient in getting it resolved.

PREVENTIVE MEASURES/CAUSES:

- Keep your pets well-groomed and parasite-free, and keep them more than paws reach away from any animal known to have mange.
- Don't breed pets with chronic conditions of mange as it is likely to be passed on to offspring. Although rarer in cats, Burmese and Siamese are more prone to mange, so be more diligent if you share your life with one of these breeds.

SIGNS & SYMPTOMS:

- Redness
- Hair loss
- Pimples
- Crusty areas
- Itchiness/Scratching

WHAT YOU MAY NEED:

A trip to the vet! Only your Veterinarian can determine which type of mange your pet has and therefore the treatment necessary. Skin scrapings and maybe a few hairs will need to be looked at under the microscope. Blood and urine tests may be taken to determine underlying conditions.

WHAT TO DO:

Follow veterinary instructions...Special dips may be in order. Launder bedding and keep your cat clean and well fed (a healthy diet means a healthier animal – mange often affects pets that are poorly nourished).

Fatty acid supplements (Omega 3s) are popular for skin disorders so discuss with your Veterinarian and often an antihistamine can help control the itch (1mg per pound of pet's body weight).

MOUTH SORES & ULCERS

CONDITION OVERVIEW:
Mouth sores can occur in older cats who have kidney or liver disease, diabetes or suffer from pancreatic tumors. They are common in cats with calicivirus (respiratory infection). They can become inflamed, be painful and prevent your pet from eating. Dental disease though too is often the culprit, but of course sores can occur anytime there is a cut, scrape or injury of any type to the mouth. Even allergies and mange around the mouth can result in sores, bumps and redness.

PREVENTIVE MEASURES/CAUSES:
- Examine your cat's mouth weekly so as to discover a small issue before it becomes a big painful problem.
- Brush your cat's teeth at least 3 times a week to prevent gingivitis, abscesses and infections. Use a pet-specific tooth brush and pet-specific tooth paste as human toothpaste can be toxic to our four-legged friends.
- Schedule regular veterinary visits but also do not hesitate to seek medical advice at the first sign of symptoms.

SIGNS & SYMPTOMS:
- Excessive drooling or panting
- Not eating or difficulty chewing
- Bad breath
- Foaming at the mouth
- Frequent gagging
- Pawing at face
- Teeth grinding
- Bloody discharge from mouth or visible sores
- Crusty nose or bleeding from the nose

WHAT YOU MAY NEED:
- Saline or purified water to clean
- Soft warm-to-cool foods (baby food)
- Anbesol®
- Saline solution

WHAT TO DO:
To treat the problem, you need the advice of your Veterinarian, but you can help to relieve some pain for your precious friend by providing a topical treatment like Anbesol® and dabbing it directly on the sore. Crushed ice or ice water may also offer temporary relief, but watch your cat -- too hot or too cold foods or liquids may be painful. Providing softer meals will allow your kitty to get his much-needed nutrition – cats often like baby food!

Follow your vet's prescribed treatment but notice any sign of infection. Rinsing her mouth with saline solution may help speed up the healing process but don't wash away beneficial medication.

Cats sometimes develop salmon-pink sores on the lips that may be mistaken for spider bites.

This may be an allergic condition called Feline Eosinophilic Granuloma Complex (aka Kitty Acne) and may also develop on the belly or backs of the thighs. Usually they are not painful but generally require veterinary assistance.

MUSCLE & JOINT INJURIES (Breaks, Sprains and Strains)

CONDITION OVERVIEW:

Since most cat parents do not have immediate access to an x-ray machine when their pet begins limping, you may not know if the animal has experienced a broken bone, muscle or tendon tear or strain. A broken bone (which requires emergency veterinary care) results when the bone cracks or actually separates due to trauma. A compound fracture (broken bone that has penetrated the skin) can cause severe bleeding and result in infection while sprains and strains occur when a ligament is over-stretched. Although painful, they often resolve on their own without surgical intervention. Should a ligament become torn, it will require surgical repair. All of these injuries are painful and can cause a great deal of swelling and distress to your kitty.

PREVENTIVE MEASURES/CAUSES:

- Keep cats fit.
- Do your best to avoid falls.
- Provide ramps in place of stairs especially for older pets. This includes getting in and out of cars, on and off sofas, beds, anywhere they could place pressure or strain joints and muscles when jumping or climbing.
- Keep cats indoors or in covered fenced yards so they will not be hit by cars.
- Small pets tossed during animal fights can suffer bone and joint injuries so keep out of harm's way.

SIGNS & SYMPTOMS:

- Acute/sudden lameness or limping accompanied by pain
- Swelling at the joint
- Scrapes or wounds around the joint due to trauma to the area
- Heat, tenderness and/or swelling at the joint
- Bone protrusion

WHAT YOU MAY NEED:

- Sam splint® or other splinting materials (rolled magazine/newspaper, popsicle sticks, unsharpened pencils, wooden spoons, bubble wrap) depending on pet's size
- Flexible conforming wrap
- Gauze squares & rolls
- Antibacterial soap
- Water
- Cold pack
- Board, towel or other means to transport pet
- Muzzle

WHAT TO DO:

If small cuts or scrapes surround the joint, gently wash with antibacterial soap to clean and pat dry. If bleeding, apply direct pressure as discussed on page 122.

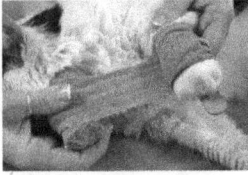

If pain level seems minimal and assumption is a slight strain, make sure your pet is confined in a small room or crate to ensure rest. Apply a cold pack to any swelling four times daily for 5-10 minute increments. Stop however if this is causing pain or distress. If not better the next day, PAWSitively see your Veterinarian.

Photo by: Sunny-dog Ink

If injury appears more serious or animal is in considerable pain, lift him into car if he will stay calm, and get veterinary assistance. If however he is anxiously moving and may cause further injury to the joint or leg, splinting may be in order:

If you suspect a break (bone penetrating skin or a limb is hanging loosely), immobilize the limb immediately by securing a popsicle stick to a cat's limb with gauze and/or self-adhering wrap. Muzzling may be important to prevent a nip. Do not attempt to apply any kind of immobilization device if the animal is resistant or in extreme pain as you could do further damage or be bitten. Seek professional veterinary help immediately.

HOMEOPATHIC TIPS: For bruising, *Arnica Montana* (Leopard's bane) is an alternative choice. It can be applied as a salve or cream or dosed as a tincture – 30c - 200c every four to twelve hours is the general starting point. Stop when you see improvement, but if there is no improvement in a few days, stop as well and obtain professional medical care.

NOSEBLEEDS

CONDITION OVERVIEW:

Known as epistaxis in the medical world, nosebleeds are not generally acute nor do they come on suddenly in cats; they may affect one or both nostrils but usually are the result of trauma due to the sensitive nasal cavities common in cats. Sometimes nosebleeds are caused by a condition known as coagulopathy, where blood just does not clot as it should. Other possibilities include wounds, an internal injury which is not visible, a tumor, cancer in an organ or Leukemia. Ingesting rat poison, injury due to a foreign object or Rocky Mountain Spotted Fever (also from ticks) may cause nosebleeds to occur.

PREVENTIVE MEASURES/CAUSES:

- Keep cats away from sharp and poisonous objects. Keep your cats tick-free.
- Do weekly head-to-tail check-ups of your cat to find problems when they are small.

SIGNS & SYMPTOMS:
- Bloody discharge from the nostrils
- Sneezing fits
- Difficulty breathing; wheezing
- Bad breath which could indicate a dental problem may be the cause

WHAT YOU MAY NEED:
- Cold compress
- Gauze squares

WHAT TO DO:
As for any injury or illness, keep your cat calm! Heavy panting or excited sneezing may exacerbate the bleeding.

Apply a cold compress and apply direct pressure with an absorbent cloth.

Never use a muzzle during a nosebleed but do try to keep cat as calm as possible so that she doesn't shake her head.

Call your Veterinarian and take your pet in if advised. Medication or even cauterization of the blood vessels may be in order as well as testing for the exact cause.

OBESITY/OVERWEIGHT

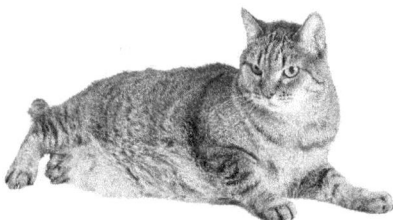

CONDITION OVERVIEW:
The Association for Pet Obesity Prevention has determined that more than half of our cats are overweight. Additionally, research shows a correlation between overweight pets and overweight owners. Fitness is important on two-legs and four-paws! Generally, lack of exercise combined with overeating is the main culprit, but there can by underlying health conditions, so start off by taking your extra fluffy feline to the Veterinarian for a check-up to make sure all systems are go for an exercise program. Even a few extra pounds increases the risk of heart disease, diabetes, respiratory illness and joint problems for your four-legged best friend and yourself, so get those paws and legs moving for a healthy lifetime together.

PREVENTIVE MEASURES/CAUSES:

- Know WHAT you are putting into your pet's body. Read cat's food labels (see pages 12-14) looking for a high quality protein as the first ingredient (unless prescribed otherwise by your Veterinarian) and low to no carbohydrates. Learn which human foods are good and which are not for your pet and get better educated on canine and feline nutrition remembering EVERY body is different and all of your pets, even if from the same litter, may not thrive on the same food. Allergies, differing metabolisms and other conditions may require every cat in the household to have a diet especially tailored to them.
- Cat Parents -- adopt yourself a second cat because nothing exercises a feline more than chasing a friend around the house! If however that is not the best choice for your living arrangement, provide Fluffy with toys and stimulation that will keep her active in addition to time with you!
- Don't miss annual check-ups at your Veterinarian. Blood tests and urinalysis may determine kidney, thyroid and other problems early and help you find a solution.

SIGNS & SYMPTOMS:
Your cat may be overweight if:

- you can't feel her ribs easily under her fur coat (you shouldn't however be able to see ribs on most breeds). On cats, the area near the base of the tail should be smooth with a slight fat covering but you should feel the bone.
- her belly hangs lower than her chest
- she doesn't have a waistline when you look down at her back from your eye level
- she has become a couch potato or tires quickly with minimal exercise

Don't use the excuse that she's not fat, just fluffy -- you are doing your cat a disservice and may be shortening her life!

WHAT YOU MAY NEED:

- There is no magic pill or quick fix! Experts will lead you on the path, so depending on the suggested course of action, you may need a new diet, exercise equipment, water therapy, etc.
- Low calorie treats -- slices of raw zucchini, apples, carrots and broccoli -- are smarter choices than fat-filled flour based biscuits.

WHAT TO DO:
First, get a good check-up at the Veterinarian for the go-ahead to begin a better exercise program. Also discuss diet and contact a feline nutritionist for the best tips and advice.

Check into the unlimited resources at your disposal but start at a speed comfortable for your cat. You too may tone up and drop a pound or two thanks to your work-out partner!

POISONING

CONDITION OVERVIEW:

Some cats spend time pouncing on the greenery – but as few as two petals or leaves from "true" lilies (Easter Lily, Tiger Lily, Day Lily and Asiatic varieties) can be fatal to our feline friends! Knowing what to do and having the necessary tools on hand can avert a minor injury or a major disaster.

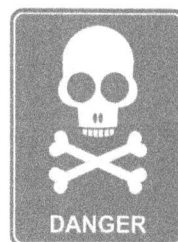

The ability for any potentially poisonous substance to cause health issues is proportional to the animal's body weight. Additionally, every item on a poison list may not harm every animal, but, if it has made the list, a significant number of animals have had an adverse reaction to it, so err on the side of caution for your cat's sake.

Cats are not small dogs! They are a different species that respond in their own unique way to food, chemicals, toxins and other creatures, including humans. Cats are glucuronidation-deficient. Glucuronidation is a metabolic process where drugs are broken down into water soluble compounds that are more easily excreted by the kidneys out of the body. What this means is that drugs stay in the feline system longer than they do in canines and they act as a higher dosage. This pertains to such medications as:

- Acetaminophen
- Aspirin
- Benzocaine
- Aricept/Donepezil
- Diazepam
- Carprofen

Cats require methods of decontamination that may differ from what we do for dogs. Particularly when it comes to emesis (induced vomiting), there are limited options for our feline friends because 1) It is very difficult to make cats vomit and 2) At home remedies can cause hemorrhagic gastritis (inflammation and painful burning sensation of the stomach).

Chocolate accounts for 50% of the calls received by the Pet Poison Helpline. It is most poisonous to dogs, cats and ferrets. Although antioxidants in dark chocolate are considered good for human hearts, the darker the chocolate, the worse it is for many animals. The culprit is theobromine -- both a cardiac stimulant and a diuretic, which can speed up the heart while pulling fluids from the body resulting in rapid heart rate and breathing, vomiting, diarrhea, seizures and even death.

One ounce of milk chocolate per pound of body weight can be fatal to our pets. The darker the chocolate, the higher the concentration of theobromine which means the less it takes to have the same ill effects.

The basic formula is below, but realize some pets are more sensitive and can be harmed by less than the amount provided on the chart:

- Milk Chocolate – 1 ounce per pound of body weight
- Dark Chocolate – ½ ounce per pound of body weight
- Baker's (unsweetened) Chocolate – ¼ ounce per pound of body weight
- Dry Cocoa Powder – 1/8 ounce (less than one teaspoon) per pound of body weight
- Cocoa Bean Mulch – Due to the variation in manufacturing, the concentration of theobromine can vary depending on the manufacturer. However, if you suspect that an animal in your care has ingested cocoa bean mulch, seek veterinary advice.

PREVENTIVE MEASURES/CAUSES:

- Every year thousands of pets needlessly suffer, and many die, from ingesting substances in our homes and even from human food. Be proactive in making sure that an animal's environment is free of potentially hazardous substances:
    - Get down on all fours and look at life from your cat's point-of-view, and also check countertops and shelves (indoors and out), and keep harmful items out of paw's and claws reach.
    - Install childproof locks on cabinet doors if you share your life with curious pets.
    - Read labels and purchase "pet friendly" chemicals and cleaners.
    - Remember that when you have a cat, you have a four-legged toddler for life.

It is your responsibility to keep your cat safe and supervise where your cat goes and what they can get into.

SIGNS & SYMPTOMS:

- Vitals not normal (see page 92)
- Rapid or decreased heart rate
- Difficulty breathing or heavy panting (which also often indicates pain)
- Slow CRT -- Shock
- Muscle tremors or seizures
- Vomiting and/or diarrhea, sometimes with blood
- Drooling or foaming
- Pawing at the mouth
- Redness of the skin, ears, eyes, any body part
- Lethargy or anxiety
- Blisters or sores on the mouth or skin where poison made contact
- Swelling
- Elevated or decreased heart rate, breathing or body temperature
- Anything that is not normal for your pet!

WHAT YOU MAY NEED:

- Phone numbers for your Veterinarian and poison control easily accessible
- ASPCA Poison Control Center Hotline (888) 426-4435
- Pet Poison Helpline (800) 213-6680 ... Fees Apply
- Know the weight of the Kitty so that you can share with your vet so that you can properly administer solutions (only on the advice of a Veterinarian).
- Water or non-fat yogurt for diluting poison

WHAT TO DO:

1. GATHER INFORMATION if you know (or suspect) that a pet has been poisoned:
   - Determine the type of poison, how much ingested and how long ago.
   - Check the animal's vital signs (temperature, heart rate, respiration, capillary refill time, gum color).
   - Observe symptoms (difficulty breathing, vomiting, diarrhea, seizures, bleeding, etc).
   - Stay calm and react to the situation in a reasonable manner. If possible, read the container label of the substance that you suspect the animal has ingested.
   - Immediately call your Veterinarian or poison control and do exactly as instructed.

2. REACT – GET TO THE VET taking cat and poison with you.

Do NOT use Hydrogen Peroxide on cats as it can inflame the stomach. In rare cases, it has proven fatal. Inducing vomiting in a cat at home should never be done! At onset of toxic ingestion, get the kitty to your closest veterinarian or animal emergency center. Dexmede-tomidine is the veterinarian's best choice yet it works only 51% of the time in cats and can be reversed with atipamezole. Xylanzine is another option, but both of these drugs have the side effect of sedation on the cat.

Other ways an animal can be poisoned:

In addition to what goes in their mouths, cats can be poisoned by toxins that are absorbed, inhaled or injected into their bodies. Therefore, knowing what, where (which body part) and how much Fluffy got into determines your course of action.

- **Absorbed poisons** are substances that get on our cat's paws and coat and are absorbed through their skin. These poisons may also be ingested once the animal licks and grooms himself.
  - Wash the area thoroughly and visit your Veterinarian to prevent long-term effects and discomfort.
  - For oil-based toxins (petroleum products), use a gentle dishwashing liquid or shampoo before flushing with water.
  - If the poison is a dry powdery substance (such as sink scrubs or granulated swimming pool chlorine), brush or vacuum away before washing the area -- if you add water to a dry toxin, you will activate it ON your pet's skin! If the irritant is in your cat's eye, carefully flush the eye with purified water/eye wash.

- **Inhaled poisons** include aerosol sprays, carbon monoxide, gases, and other fumes inhaled into your cat's lungs. Quickly get the animal into fresh air and administer rescue breathing if needed by holding her mouth shut and breathing into her nostrils – every 2-3 seconds giving tiny puff breaths.

- **Injected poisons** include insect stings and snake bites discussed in this book on pages 126 - 133.

Marijuana or cannabis poisoning (not to be confused with CBD which has beneficial properties) is on the rise with our dogs and cats with a 30% increase in calls to the Animal Poison Control Center since 2009. It can be harmful to cats and although they may become sedated and act drunk like humans, many become agitated, have increased heart rates and are in major distress. They stagger around dribbling urine and may go into a coma and die without veterinary treatment. Keep in mind that marijuana butter, brownies and cookies can be doubly dangerous with their additions of fats and chocolates. Please keep all drugs, prescribed or non-prescribed, out of paw's reach!

PLANTS
Plants are highest on the list of what cats ingest, and any plant can cause gastro-intestinal upset, even vomiting in cats. The insoluble calcium oxalate plants (calcium oxalate crystals are like tiny needles that embed themselves into the oral cavity when eaten) are most problematic and quite common as house plants. They include:
- Anthurium
- Arrowhead Vine
- Caladium
- Calla Lily
- Diffenbachia
- Peace Lily
- Philodendron
- Pothos

Wash mouth with cool water or offer tuna water or dilute chicken broth to rinse oral cavity. A diluted milk or yogurt mixture (1:1) may bind to the oxalate crystals making them less irritating to the gut. Cat may require anti-emetics and pain meds for supportive care.

Soluble CaOx plants cause irritation like the insoluble ones above but in large amounts, can cause hypocalcemia (low calcium leading to numbness, seizures, confusion and cardiac arrest) and renal issues. Plants in this category include: shamrock and edible rhubarb. With cats, get to your veterinarian to induce emesis and administer activated charcoal with sorbitol. Kidney and calcium values must be monitored and GI protectives and pain meds administered.

Lillies (sp Lilium and Hemerocallis)
ALL parts of true lilies, including the Easter Lily, are toxic to cats!
Leafy stem
Scaly bulb

Narrow leaves
6-petal flowers
Trumpet shape

Bathe cat quickly if possible, especially if pollen is on fur, mouth and any part of her body, and get her to the vet where they will induce emesis and administer activated charcoal. A CBC, Chemical Panel and UA (urinalysis) will be conducted and fluids given aggressively for 48 hours or until asymptomatic.

Pyrethrin is an insecticide derived from the Chrysanthemum flower, and Pyrethroid is a synthetic form. You may find these 'thrins' in flea control products (concentrations greater than 3% can cause problems) and due to glucuronidation, cats are very sensitive! Always take care to use cat-specific products on your kitty and if your cat co-habitates with a dog, make sure she can't rub against or lay in the same bedding if pyrethrins have been applied to the dog.

Symptoms can include
- Tremors, seizures, ataxia
- Skeletal muscle weakness

Bathe kitty with mild liquid dish soap and warm water (not too warm as to open pores allowing more of toxin to go into). If cat is twitching, she may need to be sedated at your vet's office even before bath, so act quickly.

After bath, towel dry to prevent hypothermia, keep kitty warm. Your veterinarian will need to monitor the cat for 48-72 hours, maintaining hydration and perfusion and limiting stimulus to prevent seizures.

With Amphetamine ingestion, including nasal inhalers, signs present in cats in 1-3 hours and can last for 7-34 hours. Most cats puncture tablets rather than consuming quantities like dogs, but still...GET KITTY TO THE VET! She may experience any of the following for which medically-induced emesis, activated charcoal, bloodwork will be prescribed as there is a great potential for the cat to become hypoxic (oxygen deficient) and suffer from hypoperfusion (decreased blood flow):
- Mydriasis (unusually large pupils)
- Tachycardia (increased heart beat)
- Tachypnea (rapid breathing)
- Agitation, vocalization,
- Disorientation, circling
- Hyperactivity
- Fever
- Tremors

Essential Oils

May contain terpenes rapidly absorbed orally & dermally then metabolized by liver and phenols (alcohols) are also caustic to kitties. Oil exposure can cause irritation and lesions to the tongue, mucous membranes and throat.

Oral decontamination includes diluting by administering water flavored with tuna juice to encourage drinking, pain meds, antibiotics, soft food or feeding tube if mouth and pharyngeal ulcers present, as well as oxygen support in severe cases.

Topical decontamination, most commonly cause by application of Tea Tree Oil, can result in Hypothermia, ataxia (involuntary muscle movements), Weakness, Central Nervous System depression, tremors, bradycardia (slowed heart rhythm) and increased liver enzymes.

Bathe cat well with mild hand/dish washing detergent, examining for skin irritation. It will be important for the vet to maintain hydration and perfusion, provide heat support, monitor blood pressure and administer liver protectants.

Of particular note are:

- Oil of Wintergreen and Sweet Birch (methyl salicylate) convert to aspirin causing GI & respiratory issues and anemia.
- Citrus Oil (d-limonene) may cause hypersalivation, tremors, ataxia (abnormality in muscle and eye movements – can be on just one side of the body) and coma.
- Pine oils may result in neurological and renal issues, present as vomiting, salivation, anorexia, oral and pharyngeal pain and ulcers.
- Ylang Ylang
- Peppermint Oil may cause vomiting, diarrhea, depression, seizure
- Cinnamon Oil is upsetting to gut

Bromethalin is found in rodenticides to which cats are twice as sensitive as dogs! Bromethalin ingestion cause result in Paralytic Syndrome which may last up to 8 weeks! This includes
- Hind limb weakness/ataxia, paralysis
- CNS depression
- Loss of pain
- Lack of conscious proprioception (lack of awareness of body position and movement)
- GI Stasis
- Seizures
- Coma

Xylitol, an artificial sweetener, hasn't seen significant cases in cats, according to the Pet Poison Helpline. The same holds true with grapes and raisins but you'll find both of these detrimental to the canine species

For a list of Common Household Poisons, see page 213

PROLAPSE

CONDITION OVERVIEW:
A prolapse occurs when a part of the body (typically an internal structure) slips or moves out of place generally due to trauma or illness.

PREVENTIVE MEASURES/CAUSES:
Prevent fleas, worms and other parasites from invading your cats as they could be the underlying cause of a prolapse.

Provide plenty of fresh clean water at all times to keep your cat regular and ward off urinary infections.

Areas likely to prolapse are:
- Rectum – generally caused by straining/constipation or anaphylactic shock; rectal tumors and gastrointestinal parasites may also cause this form of prolapse.
- Urethra
- Penis – inability to completely retract into the sheath (aka paraphimosis).
- Vagina (may include the uterus) – generally due to straining associated with birth (queening in cats) or vaginal hyperplasia (swelling of tissue causing protrusion through the vulva); spaying can prevent vaginal prolapse.
- Eyes – often caused from too much pressure placed above the eye socket.

SIGNS & SYMPTOMS:
- Protrusion of any body part from its normal location
- Pet may be licking or chewing at protrusion
- Pain/discomfort

WHAT YOU MAY NEED:
- K-Y® or other water soluble jelly
- Gauze
- Saline solution

WHAT TO DO:
Should you notice a protrusion, get your injured pet to prompt veterinary care. Do not try to push the protrusion back into place! The underlying cause must be determined by your Veterinarian who has the skill to then gently massage or surgically reposition the body part. Before you head out, soak gauze squares with saline solution and apply to the protruding area. This helps keep the organ's tissues from drying out and increases the chance that the Veterinarian will be able to revitalize the damaged organ tissue. Covering the body part also prevents the animal from chewing on the exposed area as does applying a cone collar to your furry patient.

When it is an eyeball that is displaced, the eyelid is curled back preventing the lid from covering the eye. Until you reach veterinary care, rinse the eye with saline every 5 minutes to prevent it from drying out.

For rectal or vaginal prolapse, you may apply water-soluble lubricating jelly to ease discomfort, but only let your Veterinarian attempt to reposition the prolapse.

In cases of paraphimosis, rinse the extruded penis with copious amounts of saline solution to help decrease inflammation of the tissues, then apply water-soluble lubricating jelly to the end. Gently moving any hairs that might be preventing retraction may allow it to return to its sheath. Medical intervention however is advised as the prepuce may constrict blood flow which could cause tissue death in the penis.

PUNCTURES & BITE WOUNDS

CONDITION OVERVIEW:
When objects pierce the skin (nails, teeth of another animal, glass, sharp sticks for instance), they leave small holes through which bacteria enters the body. Bite wounds are often disguised by fur and can develop into an abscess if they are not discovered and immediately treated. X-rays or ultrasounds might be needed to diagnose internal bleeding and damage, especially in the case of animal bites since the tearing of deep layers of muscle may have occurred. Large animals are capable of inflicting bone crushing injuries. Deep injuries around the neck and chest are commonly seen if a smaller animal is picked up and shaken by a larger one.

De-gloving injuries result when skin is torn away and include significant tissue damage and blood loss. Cats that climb into car engines suffer this injury from fan belts; dogs from animal attacks, entanglement in barbed wire fencing and even being hit by cars. If blood supply is not quickly returned to the skin, necrosis (tissue death) may occur and skin grafting may become necessary.

PREVENTIVE MEASURES/CAUSES:
- Keep your home and yard free of sharp and dangerous debris, and keep your cat out of harm's way when using garden tools, saws, grass trimmers or any machinery.
- Keep cats indoors to prevent injuries.
- Don't just sweep up broken glass…vacuum it too! Tiny shards could remain and pierce tiny paws.

SIGNS & SYMPTOMS:
- Bleeding
- Skin cut, scraped or torn away
- Puncture
- Pain
- Limping
- Licking at body parts

WHAT YOU MAY NEED:

- 4 X 4 Gauze squares
- Gauze roll
- Self-adhering compression bandage or adhesive tape
- Saline solution
- Antibacterial Soap, Chlorhexidine, Hibiclens®

WHAT TO DO:

Stop bleeding by applying direct pressure. If the wound is not bleeding, rinse with saline solution or antibacterial soap. Puncture wounds that penetrate all layers of the skin can allow bacteria to penetrate deeply into the body. As the tissue begins to close, the bacteria can quickly get trapped and cause infection, so get to your Veterinarian.

If the puncture is from an animal bite, find out if other animal is current on her vaccinations (if possible). Pain, redness and infection can occur around untreated areas and your pet may develop a fever, loss of appetite and become lethargic. Antibiotics most likely will be needed to get her through this episode.

Punctures to the Chest (Sucking Chest Wounds)

CONDITION OVERVIEW:

The cavity inside your cat's chest normally allows the lungs to easily expand when air is inhaled. However, when an object protrudes the chest wall, air gets sucked into the chest cavity and that pressure collapses the lungs, preventing them from expanding and resulting in suffocation. This sort of injury, caused by a bite or piercing object (including a knife, bullet, arrow, stick or even a broken rib), is commonly called a sucking wound because of the way air is pulled into the hole made by the object. Even if nothing appears to have punctured an animal's chest, if you hear a gurgling sound and/or see frothy blood, something (most likely a rib) has penetrated. *You have a life-threatening emergency to help your pet through. You must get veterinary help but following the "What To Do" steps below can help...*

PREVENTIVE MEASURES/CAUSES:

- Do your best to keep cats out of harm's way...NEVER allow them where hunting or even recreational sporting events take place. Bullets, arrows and even BB guns can fatally wound or seriously injure your cat.
- Keep pets safe when working with yard equipment. Rocks and other debris can fly out of lawnmowers and grass trimmers causing puncture injuries.
- Only allow your cat around other animals you know and watch out for wildlife. Don't let pets roam freely, especially at nighttime. It only takes seconds for the worst to happen.
- If a cat has been hit by a car or struck in the chest, assume she could have a sucking wound to the chest (possibly due to a broken rib penetrating the lung), so quickly and carefully assess and get professional help.

SIGNS & SYMPTOMS:
- Bubbling of blood at chest site
- Slow breathing or fast and labored
- Abdomen may move more with each breath
- Animal may try stretching neck to facilitate breathing

WHAT YOU MAY NEED:
- Gauze squares
- Gauze rolls
- K-Y Jelly® or other water soluble gel
- Honey or Karo® syrup
- Plastic wrap
- Adhesive tape or self-adhering wrap
- Towels/blankets

WHAT TO DO:
Your goal is to make a one-way valve that prevents air from being sucked into the chest cavity. You want to re-establish the normal "vacuum" that should exist in the cavity, prevent lung collapse and help pet breathe easy until medical help is available.

1) Treat your cat for shock (see page 188) after checking CRT (page 92). Keep her warm and put a drop or two of honey or Karo® Syrup on her gums.

2) If the wound has a small opening, seal it with a big glob of K-Y Jelly® to prevent incoming air from collapsing the lung.

3) Place clean gauze or plastic wrap (even a plastic baggie will suffice) on top of the opening and hold in place with tape on 3 of the 4 sides. When the animal inhales, his lungs will push air out of the chest cavity and back through the hole, so your bandaging will need to lift on that one side to release air from the body. When the animal exhales, and the lungs deflate, the sucking wound will pull the plastic back against the hole and prevent additional air from entering the chest and collapsing the lung.

4) If the wound is too large for water soluble lubricating jelly, cover tightly with plastic wrap to form a seal and tape it in place. If possible, have the kitty lie on the injured side to keep pressure on the bleeding and help seal the hole.

5) *Get Immediate Veterinary Attention.*

REVERSE SNEEZE

CONDITION OVERVIEW:
Known as Inspiratory Paroxysmal Respiration or Pharyngeal Gag Reflex, a reverse sneeze comes on suddenly and causes the cat to extend his head and neck while making rapid inspiratory movements (inhalations), generally with his mouth closed causing "snorting" sounds to come from the nasal passages. Often referred to as a backward sneeze in which irritation causes the soft palate to spasm, it may be due to irritation in the sinuses but most often remains a mystery, even to the most competent Veterinarians. Cats are less likely to have this condition so if your kitty does, have her checked out by your Veterinarian as some felines are prone to an asthma-type condition which dogs are not.

PREVENTIVE MEASURES/CAUSES:
- None really but provide a dust-free environment for any cat prone to this ailment.
- Have your Veterinarian check-out your cat to rule out certain underlying causes.

SIGNS & SYMPTOMS:
- Rapid and long inspirations (inhaling) resulting in a loud snorting sound.
- Dog stands still and may extend his head and/or neck forward as the trachea may have narrowed during the spasm and he is trying to get more air.

WHAT YOU MAY NEED:
- Patience. Episodes generally subside in a matter of minutes, but stand by in case this is only the beginning to a bigger problem.

WHAT TO DO:
Encourage your cat to drink water, but do not force her to.

Most cats just need the spasm to run its course of 20-30 seconds to several minutes.

Once the sneezing stops, most pets return to normal with no ill effects. If yours does not however, seek veterinary care after immediately checking vitals (including capillary refill time) and making sure he is breathing. It's often a good idea to video an episode to show your Veterinarian for confirmation as you'll never get your kitty to have a reverse sneeze on command in the doctor's office!

SECONDHAND SMOKE

CONDITION OVERVIEW/PRECAUTIONS:
Tobacco smoke exhaled by humans plus the actual smoke released from a pipe, burning cigarette or cigar contains thousands of chemicals including harmful ones like carbon monoxide, arsenic, formaldehyde and benzene. The last several decades have proven that people who are repeatedly exposed to environmental tobacco smoke are more likely to develop lung cancer, breathing and heart problems than those who are not exposed to these chemicals. Recent studies show similar findings in our companion pets citing increased eye irritation, lung and nasal cancers in cats who cohabitate with human smokers and who are subject to chronic exposure.

PREVENTIVE MEASURES/CAUSES:
- Make sure your cat has a clean sleeping and living environment. If you smoke, do so outside where it can dissipate and not linger where you cat lives and breathes.
- Make sure cigar and cigarettes and their discarded butts are kept out of paw's and claws reach.
- An air purifier may help rid your home of harmful impurities for you and your cat, smoke or not. Antioxidants, such as vitamin C, can rid the body of some free-radicals.

SIGNS & SYMPTOMS:
- Red, irritated eyes (may paw at them)
- Raspy breaths; difficulty breathing
- Coughing, gasping sounds
- Coughing up blood or blood coming from nasal passages

WHAT YOU MAY NEED:
- Veterinary check-up!

WHAT TO DO:
Get to the Veterinarian and follow recommended treatment.

SEIZURES & CONVULSIONS

CONDITION OVERVIEW:

A seizure or convulsion is a sudden excessive firing of nerves in the brain that results in a series of involuntary muscle contractions and abnormal behaviors lasting from seconds to minutes. Severity can range from a glazed-over look in the eyes to twitching in a part of the face to the animal falling on his side, barking, gnashing his teeth, urinating, defecating and running in place while lying down. Seizures are symptoms of poisoning or a neurological disorder and are not in themselves a disease.

PREVENTIVE MEASURES/CAUSES:

- Some seizures are idiopathic meaning the cause cannot be determined, but others are results of:
- Poisoning (chocolate or snail/slug bait pellets for instance)
- Low blood sugar
- Brain tumor or head trauma
- Liver disease
- Inflammation or an infectious disease of the nervous system
- Epilepsy (when all else is ruled out, this is the general diagnosis)
- Stress or extreme anxiety

SIGNS & SYPMTOMS:

The 3 Stages of a Seizure

- **Aura** is the first stage and may occur seconds before to several days prior to a seizure. Restlessness, whining/crying, shaking, salivation, wandering aimlessly, hiding or even overly needy or affectionate signs may by demonstrated by your cat.
- **Ictus** is when the seizure occurs. You may notice a glazing over of the eyes and staring just as it is about to occur. We refer to this as "the lights are on, but nobody is home" look.
- **Postictal** is the stage immediately following the seizure when the cat appears confused, disoriented and may be unresponsive. Animal may not have great control of motor skills or bodily functions and may need assistance getting up or walking and may stumble or easily fall.

WHAT YOU MAY NEED:

- Stop watch to time seizure
- A calm demeanor as your emotional state, and that of those around you, may affect the patient
- Baby gate (if this is an ongoing situation for your cat, you'll want to make sure she can't tumble down stairs and you may want to leave your cat confined in a room when you can't supervise her.)

WHAT TO DO:

Once a seizure starts, there is nothing you can do to stop it. The goal is to keep the kitty from injuring itself.

- If other animals are in the vicinity, get them behind a closed door away from the seizing pet. Many animals, even the gentlest and most obedient, will attack a seizing animal as the seizure appears to them to be an act of aggression.
- Stay away from animal's mouth. During a seizure the cat will not be in voluntary control of its actions. However, the jaws perform involuntary muscle contractions, and if you get in the way, teeth will meet flesh.
- *Think CALM & COMFORTABLE or SOFT & SERENE*, whichever terms resonate with you.

   Toss SOFT/COMFORTABLE blankets or pillows around the animal for cushioning, especially if the seizure is happening on a hard surface; remove tables and chairs from next to the pet.

   Stay CALM and create a SERENE environment by reducing noise, anxiety and stimulation of any type (turn off televisions and stereo components, dim lights, close draperies over bright windows and remove angst-filled humans, and other animals from the area).

- Time the seizure (all three stages if possible). If this is a first-time seizure or unusually long for your epileptic pet, have her checked out by your Veterinarian. If multiple seizures are occurring in a 24-hour period, also get immediate veterinary help.

Never leave a cat that has just experienced a seizure alone. If you have a cat prone to seizures that is home alone during parts of the day, make sure she stays in a safe room… free of sharp/hard corners and places she could get trapped in or fall from if disoriented. Install baby gates near stairways or even where there are only a few steps to prevent injuries.

SHOCK

CONDITION OVERVIEW:

Shock is a life-threatening condition that occurs when your pet does not get sufficient blood flow and oxygen to his tissues and organs. The body tries to compensate by increasing the heart and respiratory rates, restricting urinary output to maintain fluids and constricting blood vessels near the skin. All this requires additional energy the animal doesn't have since his vitals are not functioning properly and will result in death without quick medical care. Hypovolemic shock is when severe blood and fluid loss render the heart unable to pump sufficient blood to the body. Neurogenic shock, caused by a relaxation of muscles, causes blood pressure to drop and is usually the result of a severe spinal injury or electrocution.

PREVENTIVE MEASURES/CAUSES:

Know your cat! Causes of shock may include heart failure, sepsis (blood infection), anaphylactic shock, traumatic injury, dehydration and blood loss. When your cat does not appear right, immediately look at his gum color and check CRT (page 92) to determine if treatment for Shock is a priority!

SIGNS & SYMPTOMS:
- Capillary Refill Time exceeds 2 seconds (see page 92)
- Pet appears woozy or weak; as if over-exerted
- Panting
- Rapid heart rate
- Bright red gums

Late stage signs of shock include:
- Pale skin and gums – slow CRT (Capillary Refill Time)
- Drop in body temperature – cold extremities
- Slow respiratory rate
- Weak or absent pulse
- Depression or apathy
- Unconsciousness

WHAT YOU MAY NEED:
- Towel or blanket
- Honey or Karo Syrup®
- Electrolyte Solution (1/2 tsp salt, ½ tsp baking soda, 2 cups water)
- Immediate transport to Veterinarian

WHAT TO DO:
- Check capillary refill time (CRT) by pressing on the cats gum. If it takes more than two seconds for pink color to return to gums (or if the gums are too pale to evaluate CRT), the animal may be experiencing shock.
- Elevate kitty's hind quarters slightly by placing a pillow or folded blanket underneath to increase circulation. Do not elevate if you suspect a broken back or if there is a bleeding head or chest injury. In that case, lie flat or elevate area of wound if bleeding is heavy.
- Retain cat's body heat by covering her with a sheet or blanket, including a blanket underneath if surface beneath her is cold such as a tile floor, concrete or even the ground.
- Gently rub pet's gums with honey or Karo Syrup® to get glucose to the brain.
- Transport to a veterinary hospital immediately. Always call ahead to be assured they can accommodate you and that they are ready to help. Check ahead to see if you should administer electrolytes on the way (1/2 tsp per 30 lbs. of body weight every 30 minutes).

SKIN ALLERGIES & INFECTIONS

CONDITION OVERVIEW:
The skin is the body's first line of defense. It protects your cat from the outside elements including micro-organisms, prevents moisture loss and keeps her body thermo-regulated. Slightly thinner than our human skin, your cat's skin covers the blood and lymphatic vessels, nerves, sweat and sebaceous glands and hair follicles and is considered the largest organ of their body. It therefore goes through wear and tear and is subjected to bacteria, fungi and parasites as well as cuts and abrasions. Hormonal imbalances too can result in skin changes. Cats can suffer from red, itchy, oily or flaky skin with or without hair loss to the area. Although medical treatment is often necessary to cure the problem, a great first step can be making your pet more comfortable. Scratching and chewing are amongst the biggest summertime complaints pet owners share with their Veterinarians. Skin allergies (which can lead to infections) are generally caused by either fleas (or other parasites/insects), food or environment (grass, pollens, chemicals on floors, bedding or lawns). They result in non-stop itching, scratching and then open sores that take forever to heal. Masking the itch may help your kitty find relief, but getting to the underlying cause is the only way to break this vicious and uncomfortable cycle.

PREVENTIVE MEASURES/CAUSES:
Bathe your cat frequently. Confer with your Veterinarian and Groomer to determine how often: 1-2 times per month may be necessary to remove yeast and keep your pet's skin clean. A good brushing several times per week can help remove dirt and distribute oils evenly throughout your pet's skin and coat.

Perform a weekly Head-to-Tail check-up (page 37) so that you can more readily find a small scrape, a burr or foxtail or any sign of problem on your best friend.

Use monthly parasite preventives to keep fleas, ticks and the resulting allergies and bacteria at bay. Even if you don't see fleas, it doesn't mean they are not biting your four-legged friend. Get out a flea comb (tiny close together tines or teeth) and brush at the base of your pet's tail. If you get tiny dark specks, place them on a damp paper towel and if it turns pink... those specs are, in fact, flea dirt containing the dried blood of your pet! Some cats can develop an allergy after only a few bites, so use the monthly flea preventive your Veterinarian recommends and use it according to instructions -- pet's body weight, species (never dog meds on cats for instance) and frequency.

Other cats develop hypersensitivities to components in their diets. Many cats no longer tolerate fish or chicken. Feline and canine nutritionists (experts trained beyond the level of most Veterinarians in regards to a pet's diet) are recommending novel (new) proteins such as lamb, venison and ostrich. A diagnosis requires food trials so you may need to start eliminating an ingredient every few weeks from your pet's diet to determine what is causing the negative reaction. If the itching subsides, you have determined the ingredient that doesn't work with Fluffy's system. You can slowly add some of those ingredients back in, one at a time, and if the itching reoccurs, you've determined the culprit!

As for the environment, grass, weeds, pollen, mold spores, dust mites, fertilizers, insecticides, carpet powder and laundry detergent can irritate your pet and make him scratch his paws off. Intradermal tests can be performed at your Veterinarian's office. Although cortisone and/or steroid injections may ease the itch, knowing what is causing it and keeping it away from your pet is the best solution. A good old-fashioned oatmeal bath and calamine lotion may help him find relief in the meantime, and adding fatty acids to your pet's diet (fish oils/coconut oil) can be a solve or at least a help.

SIGNS & SYMPTOMS:
- Constant licking and chewing of paws or any body part
- Skin is red with or without a foul smell
- Patches of hair may be missing

WHAT YOU MAY NEED:
- Gentle bacterial soap or oatmeal bath
- Calamine lotion
- Aloe vera gel
- Blunt-nosed scissors
- Cone collar to prevent licking/scratching
- Benadryl® (not containing Cetirizine, Acetaphetamine or Pseudoephedrine) or medication prescribed by your Veterinarian

WHAT TO DO:
Cleanse the area with warm water and a mild (non-stinging) anti-bacterial soap or oatmeal shampoo. Rinsing with cooled chamomile or calendula tea may bring relief from itchiness.

Clip hair short with blunt-nosed scissors if it hinders a good examination. Using a razor may irritate the skin and hurt your pet. Applying calamine lotion or aloe vera gel may sooth the itch but is not a long-term fix. You need to determine the source.

Try treatment for hot spots (page 167) if the area seems to be staying too moist, but truly an examination by your Veterinarian is in order to determine the cause.

1 mg Benadryl® per every pound of your cat's body weight might make her sleepy enough to stop scratching until she reaches the veterinary office, but check first to confirm that it won't interfere with any testing that will need to be performed, medications your pet is taking or conditions your pet may have. . Also make sure Benedryl® does not contain cetirizine, acetaphenomine or pseudoephedrine.

HOMEOPATHIC TIP: For allergic dermatitis and other rashes, *Rhus Toxicodenodron* may help the body alleviate symptoms. Realize that most chronic skin conditions are related to diet. Tonic herbs support your pet's system in de-toxifying allowing her to heal herself. A good basic formula is:

2 parts burdock root, 1 part dandelion, 1 part red clover and 1 part garlic powder steeped in water and cooled and fed 1 tablespoon daily per 40 lbs. of your pet's body weight. Flax, fish oil or omega-3s should also be fed daily.

TOAD POISONING

CONDITION OVERVIEW:

Amphibians secrete a mucus through their skin to help them evade predators, but in some species this slime is toxic and can cause harm to your pet if ingested or absorbed through his skin. The Colorado River Toad (found west of the Pecos River in Southern California and the Southwestern part of the United States) and the Marine Toad (found in Hawaii and from Corpus Christi, Texas, east down the Gulf Coast into Florida) can actually kill your precious pet! The toxins can affect the heart and nervous system and lead to death.

PREVENTIVE MEASURES/CAUSES:

- Teach your cat to "leave it" and not chase after critters. Better yet, keep her indoors away from temptation.
- Always be right by her side when investigating new and uncharted territory where creatures inhabit.

SIGNS & SYMPTOMS:

- Long strings of saliva coming from your pet's mouth
- Seizures
- Collapse

WHAT YOU MAY NEED:

- Water to rinse your cat's mouth
- Transportation to get your kitty to help

WHAT TO DO:

Toad poisoning is a true medical emergency. Rinse your pet's mouth with water using a spray bottle for several minutes and get him to the Veterinarian keeping a watch on his vitals en route! Lean your cat's head forward or to the side, spraying so that the water drains out the mouth rather than being swallowed since you are rinsing away a toxin.

Should he demonstrate signs of shock, cardiac or pulmonary arrest, refer to those pages in this book to get you through until you reach veterinary care.

TONGUE SWELLING

CONDITION OVERVIEW:

A swollen tongue is most often a result of an allergic reaction due to bee stings, medication, food or an embedded object. Tongue swelling can be serious as it may prevent your kitty from eating or even interfere with his breathing (as in the case of electrocution!) *Medical treatment is a must*, but there are a few things you can do to reduce suffering and maybe even save your cat's life!

PREVENTIVE MEASURES/CAUSES:

- Get down on all fours to regularly observe your pet's environment from her perspective so that you can find sharp, toxic and dangerous objects before she does.
- Teach pets to "leave it" around bees as well as electric cords. Secure wires or unplug them in rooms where cats are left alone.
- When giving new medications, be available to observe your cat for several hours after the first dose or two to make sure she doesn't have a negative reaction.

SIGNS & SYMPTOMS:

- Difficulty breathing or difficulty closing mouth
- Red and/or swollen tongue
- Drooling
- Not willing to eat or drink

WHAT YOU MAY NEED:

- Cool water
- Tweezers, gauze square or gloved fingers to remove item
- Benadryl® (not containing Cetirizine, Acetaphetamine or Pseudoephedrine) if bee sting related

WHAT TO DO:

Offer cool water to your pet to alleviate discomfort and swelling.

Check for foreign object in your pet's mouth if he will let you do so without harm to yourself. Grasp his tongue with a piece of gauze and with your fingers or tweezers, remove the object. It is best to have someone else available to hold your pet while you do this.

If you suspect the swelling is due to a caustic or toxic substance, use a squirt or spray bottle with water to dilute the effects. Lean your cat's head forward or to the side, spraying so that the water drains out the mouth rather than being swallowed since you may be rinsing away a toxin.

If the swelling is due to a bee sting (see pages 126-128), an antihistamine might serve him best – 1mg Benedryl® per pound of your pet's body weight and monitor him closely for any additional reactions. If the swelling persists or any other symptoms such as labored breathing present themselves, get to the Veterinarian at once.

TOOTH LOSS OR DAMAGE

CONDITION OVERVIEW:
Periodontal disease (inflamed gums) is the most common reason for loss of an adult tooth in a cat. Bacteria in plaque damages the gums and connective tissue around the base of the tooth resulting in inflammation and tooth loss. A metabolic disorder known as hyperparathyroidism could also be the culprit as it reduces calcium from bones and teeth leading to tooth loss. That said, trauma (a fall or blow to the face) or chewing on hard materials (especially when getting a stick or other sharp object caught between teeth) can also result in tooth loss or damage and requires veterinary care.

PREVENTIVE MEASURES/CAUSES:
- Avoid letting your cat chew on hard items that could snap her teeth.
- Practice good dental care by brushing your cat's teeth 3-4 times weekly and getting annual veterinary exams.

SIGNS & SYMPTOMS:
- Bleeding, swelling, redness
- Drooling
- Not eating

WHAT YOU MAY NEED:
- Milk
- Cool Water
- Anbesol®
- Cotton-tipped swabs

WHAT TO DO:
Preserve any knocked-out teeth by placing them in a container of milk to protect the tissue and keep moist.

Offer your kitty cool water to diminish pain and swelling and get him to the Veterinarian.

DO NOT use Anbesol® on cats -- the active ingredient Benzocaine is toxic to cats! Although sometimes prescribed for dogs, remember; canine, feline and human bodies are different.

Provide soft food while your cat's mouth heals.

UNDER WEIGHT (Anorexia)

CONDITION OVERVIEW:
Some cats are finicky eaters, but this can be a concern for any pet parent whose furry kid is considerably underweight. You should be able to feel the ribs but not see them. If ribs and hip bones are prominent, speak with your Veterinarian.

PREVENTIVE MEASURES/CAUSES:
- Problems with teeth or gums
- Stomach issues
- Sense of smell waning
- Stress/change in environment

SIGNS & SYMPTOMS:
- Not eating
- Vomiting
- Weight loss/ribs showing, eyes sunken, hair loss

WHAT YOU MAY NEED:
- Nutrient dense food prescribed by Veterinarian and supplemental vitamins

WHAT TO DO:
First, get a veterinary check-up for blood testing and to determine any underlying causes, then follow your medical professional's instructions.

If it's an older cat who may have lost their sense of smell, warming food could increase aroma and stimulate appetite, as can adding strong smelling fish oils (omega 3s).

HOMEOPATHIC TIP: If anorexia is not linked to any underlying illness, 1 30c of Alfalfa per 20 lbs. of your pet's body weight 4 times daily may increase appetite.

URINARY BLOCKAGE

CONDITION OVERVIEW:
This is a more common condition in males as the urethra (the tube draining urine from the bladder) in your female cat is wider and allows stones (inflammatory material that forms in the kidneys due to viral infections or diet) to more readily pass. When stones create a blockage, pressure increases in the upper urinary tract and the kidneys fail. Waste then builds up making the blood toxic and results in death if quick medical action is not taken.

PREVENTIVE MEASURES/CAUSES:
- Cats, generally, require less as they generally derive most of their water from their food but should still drink at least 4-6 ounces of water a day, especially if they are not on a moist-food diet.
- Some cats prefer to drink from mugs, glasses or bowls from which their whiskers don't touch the sides.

SIGNS & SYMPTOMS:
- Straining to urinate
- More frequent need -- cat runs to litter box with no output
- Inappropriate urination (in places they usually would not go) as they can't make it to the correct place in time
- Blood or dark fluid in the urine
- Distended lower abdomen, usually painful to the touch
- Cats may go into hiding
- Later stages include loss of appetite, sluggishness and vomiting

WHAT YOU MAY NEED:
- Your observation skills -- tune in to your cat to notice her habits and react when they change.

WHAT TO DO:
Call your Veterinarian immediately if you notice your cat isn't releasing urine on a regular schedule. This can be excruciating to your cat and can be deadly since toxins that can't be voided end up in the blood stream and travel to the organs and tissues.

VOMITING (Emesis) ---- (see Diarrhea page 153)

WORMS

CONDITION OVERVIEW:
A large percentage of kittens are born with roundworms/ascarids that they received through their momma's milk. Female roundworms can produce 200,000 eggs per day so they can quickly obstruct your pet's intestines. Whipworms & hookworms are seen more frequently in dogs than in cats. Tapeworms get inside your cat if they ingest a flea as fleas find tapeworm eggs to be quite tasty. Tapeworms are made up of segments that when eliminated from your pet's body look like a grain of wiggling rice in his feces or around his anus.

PREVENTIVE MEASURES/CAUSES:

- Get kittens promptly de-wormed or at the first sign of worms in the feces or a bloated kitty belly (most need it by 4 weeks and several times until 6 months of age.)
- Apply species-specific, weight-appropriate flea treatment to keep these parasites away from your pet.

SIGNS & SYMPTOMS:

- Butt scooting and/or licking at backside
- White segments, blood or mucus in stool
- Pot-bellied appearance in kittens
- Weight-loss
- Fatigue
- Visual identification of a roundworm or tapeworm

WHAT YOU MAY NEED:

Anthelmintics are medications that expel or destroy parasitic worms without harm to the dog or cat. Your Veterinarian needs to prescribe the type needed and proper dosage so give exactly as recommended.

WHAT TO DO:

Take a stool sample to your Veterinarian so that he or she can determine which type of worm your cat has and how to best eliminate the pesky parasite before it becomes a bigger issue.

NOTE: Heartworm disease in cats is very different from heartworm disease in dogs. The cat is an atypical host for heartworms, and most worms in cats do not survive to the adult stage. Cats with adult heartworms typically have just one to three worms, and many cats affected by heartworms have no adult worms.

While this means heartworm disease often goes undiagnosed in cats, it's important to understand that even immature worms cause real damage in the form of a condition known as heartworm associated respiratory disease (HARD).

Moreover, the medication used to treat heartworm infections in dogs cannot be used in cats, so ***prevention is the only means of protecting cats*** from the effects of heartworm disease.

SIGNS & SYMPTOMS:

Initially none are observed but eventually...

- Coughing
- Easily winded
- Unconsciousness from lack of blood getting to brain
- Abnormal lung sounds
- Fluid retention

NOTES:

NOTES:

First-Aid Conclusion

Hopefully you now feel much more confident and prepared to help a cat in your care. Knowing the skills is important, but developing the confidence to calmly and effectively react is essential to your cat's chances for recovery.

Please, please, please familiarize yourself further with this material BEFORE you need it, and practice as many of the techniques as you can. It is perfectly safe and advisable to practice muzzling and bandaging on the family cat and is important for them to become comfortable with you doing so. Just take care to cause no discomfort and never leave a muzzled pet unattended. If the first time your cat is muzzled or bandaged happens to be when she is truly injured and in pain, your task will be much more difficult and your pet's stress level will be off the charts. If she knows these tools go on and then come off from time spent practicing with you, things will go much more smoothly for you both when you actually need to accomplish the techniques. In other words…the first time you practice your skills should not be during an actual emergency!

Do not however attempt to perform a choking maneuver or CPCR on a healthy cat (feel free to try on a stuffed cat though) or do not give any medications if not warranted.

Read this material, practice, re-read and practice some more so that knowing what to do becomes second nature for both you and your four-legged patient. Then should the worst happen…you will feel confident enough to react quickly so that the two of you can safely arrive at your Veterinarian with the best possible chances for a great outcome!

It's always better to have skills and knowledge and not need them than to need them and not have them!

Paws & fingers crossed for a happy lifetime together!

There is always more to learn and it should be every cat guardian's priority to continue to learn and grow. This book serves as a strong foundation from which to build your pet care knowledge. Still, there is so much more that the authors and publisher would have loved to added to this book. All involved made it their mission to provide and prepare pet guardians for common and uncommon situations that they may encounter.

One Final Important Reminder:

Important Note Regarding Cat Care, First-Aid & CPCR Techniques Provided In This Book

If you have any questions about your pet's health, seek professional veterinary care immediately!

These instructions and the contents of this book are designed to help you keep your cat more comfortable and aid with minor problems when you are unable to get to (or are on your way to) an animal hospital.

They are not meant to be a substitute for care by a licensed veterinary professional.

No liability is assumed by the authors, publisher or any other party with respect to the information, suggestions and techniques described in this book.

Should there be any discrepancy between the suggestions offered and the advice of a Veterinarian who has knowledge of the pet in question, it is recommended that the advice of the Veterinarian be followed since the Veterinarian has the advantage of physically examining the cat and knowing its medical history and circumstances.

ABOUT THE AUTHORS

DENISE FLECK

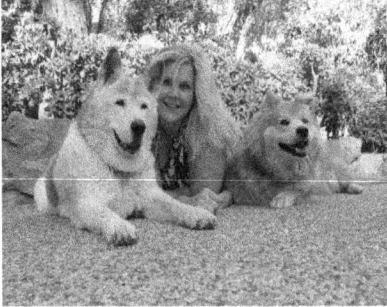

Photo by: Richard Oshen

Denise Fleck developed the curriculum for her Pet First-Aid & CPCR Classes after training with a dozen national organizations, taking seminars to this day about everything animal, reading, practicing and serving as a long-time rescue volunteer and animal response team member. She has personally taught more than 20,000 humans animal life-saving skills and millions more via on-air demonstrations. She assisted Homeland Security with their K9 Border Patrol First-Aid Program and developed her own line of Pet First-Aid Kits because "My students have the best of intentions but just don't get around to getting them together themselves." Denise has shared animal life-saving skills on Animal Planet's "Groomer Has It" and "Pit Boss", A&E's "Kirstie Alley's Big Life", CBS-TV's "The Doctors", CNN Headline News, PBS-TV's "Lassie's Pet Vet" and KTLA Los Angeles as well as on radio and in magazines.

Denise has also created the curriculum for and teaches a 20 week course in Animal Care through the Burbank Unified School District's ROP Program for high school juniors & seniors at the Burbank Animal Shelter. "My proudest moment is when one student shared that he now wants to save an animal's life rather than fighting dogs like his friends. That is why I do what I do! As the proud instructor, I hope one of my students will cure a debilitating canine disease or end animal homelessness, but if each student adopts a shelter pet, shares with friends the need for spay/neuter, never harms or judges a dog by his breed alone, I'll still wag my tail."

Her other books include *The Autumn Winter of Your Pet: Make Those Senior Years Golden, The Pet Safety Crusader's My Pet & Me Guide to Pet Disaster PAWparedness, Quickfind Books Dog First Aid & CPR, Cat First Aid & CPR, How to Take Care of Your Dog or Puppy and How to Take Care of Your Cat or Kitten; Rescue Critters Pet First Aid for Kids* and her award-winning *Don't Judge a Book by its Cover* which received the Dog Writers Association of America's Maxwell Medallion for Best Children's Book of 2014 and first sequel, "Start off on the Right Paw". Denise has also won 2 MUSE Awards and 2 Special Awards from the Cat Writer's Association, 5 Maxwell Medallions from the Dog Writer's Association, Volunteer of the Year from the Burbank Police Department for her work at the Animal Shelter and has twice been a finalist as the Pet Industry's Woman of the Year.

Denise and her husband Paul live with two rescued Akitas, Haiku & Bonsai.

Learn more at www.PetSafetyCrusader.com.

ROBERT SEMROW

Robert Semrow, like so many other pet parents, was rescued by two wonderful and amazing dogs that changed his life in ways few could imagine. Sugar and Zoey were truly special beings that changed Robert's direction in life. Sugar's special needs inspired Robert to create The Pawtographer, www.thepawtographer.com.

From there, Robert founded Pet World Insider, and then Pet World Media Group, a media company focused on the pet world. Robert's love and passion for the pet world led him to become deeply involved in many areas of the pet world from pet nutrition to pet safety and much more. Robert has interviewed, worked with and learned from many of the best and brightest in the pet world. His passion for the pet world is only matched by his desire to learn and share what he learns with fellow pet parents.

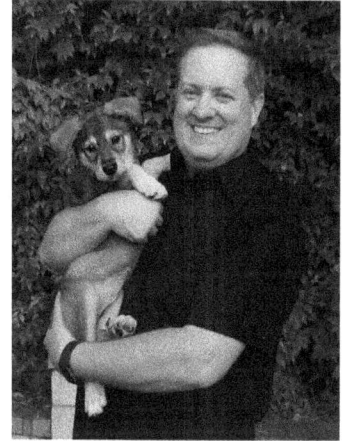

Robert has shared his knowledge, expertise and passion for the pet world on national television programs, via new media outlets and also on AM/FM/XM radio stations across North America. He has shared expertise on pet health, nutrition, behavior and more with audiences around the world. One of his greatest pleasures and missions is to learn and share what he learns.

Robert resides in Southern California with his wife, Amber, his daughters Amaya and Aubrey, and his beloved pets Bella Gem, Hatch and Faith.

Learn more about Robert and his projects at www.petworldinsider.com

PART III - RESOURCES

Pet Disaster PAWparedness Checklist
Pet's Health Record
Cat Head-to-Tail Chart
Healthy Cat Weight Chart
Body Language Visual Chart
Body Language Description Chart
Poisonous Plant chart
Common Poisons List
Missing Pet Flyer
Pet Vitals Chart
Pet Emergency ID Card
Pet Alert Information

PAWparedness Check List
for _____

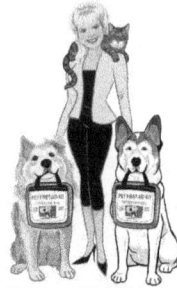

- ☐ **Properly fitting Collar, Harness, Leash & Muzzle**
- ☐ **Crate / Carrier, Stakes / Tie-out**
- ☐ **Extra ID Tags**
- ☐ **Food (use by date _____)**
- ☐ **Water**
- ☐ **Medications / Supplements including instructions and any care / behavioral needs**
- ☐ **Bowls, spoon & can Opener**
- ☐ **Grooming Supplies (wipes, brushes, combs, clippers, etc...)**
- ☐ **Clean-Up Bags, Disposable Litter Pan, Litter & Scoop**
- ☐ **Species-specific needs**
- ☐ **Blankets / Bedding / Toys (shirt that smells like YOU)**
- ☐ **Pet Medical Records / Proof of Vaccinations**
- ☐ **Pictures of all pets with all family members (include identifying features)**
- ☐ **Disinfectant, Paper Towels, Soap**
- ☐ **Plastic Bags, Zip Ties, Duct Tape**
- ☐ **Pet First Aid Kit**
- ☐ **Flash Light**
- ☐ **Transistor Radio**
- ☐ **Human Supplies & First Aid Kit**

VIP Names & Numbers:
Veterinarian: _____
Animal ER: _____
Pet Sitter / Designated Caregiver #1: _____
Pet Sitter / Designated Caregiver #2: _____
Police: _____
Fire: _____

Directions To Our House & Our Phone Number:
_____
_____

www.SunnyDogInk.com

MY PET'S HEALTH RECORD

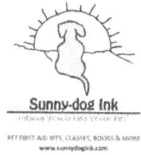

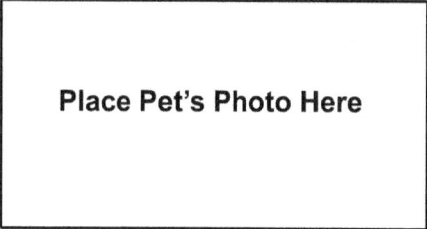

Sunny-dog Ink

Date Updated: _____

Pet's Name: _____

Pet's Sex: _____   Birth Date: _____

Species: _____   Breed: _____

Weight: _____   Color(s): _____

Special Markings: _____

Normal Temperature: _____   Normal Pulse: _____   Normal Respiration: _____

Microchip #: _____   Phone Number For Microchip Agency: _____

Vaccinations: _____
_____
_____

Veterinarian: _____   Phone Number: _____

Address & Directions: _____
_____

Animal Emergency Center: _____   Phone Number: _____

Address & Directions: _____
_____

Diet: _____

Medications & Supplements: _____
_____

Daily Exercise: _____

Sleeping Location: _____

Recent Medical History: _____
_____

Place Pet's Photo Here

CAT

Knowing what is normal for your pet can help you determine what is not!

WEEKLY "HEAD-TO-TAIL CHECK-UP" WORKSHEETS FOR CATS

Use this worksheet to note any bumps, lumps, irregularities, scars or surgeries your cat has.

Use a different color pen to note changes you find (size, color, smell, sensitivity etc.) and report them to your Veterinarian.

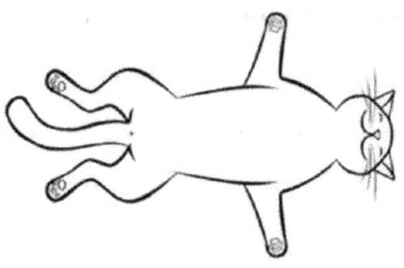

Belly

Back

Skin
Coat / Overall appearance
Crown / Skull
Eyes / Pupils
Ears
Muzzle
Snout
Mouth
Teeth
Gums / Check capillary refill time _____
Neck
Hydration
Chest / Ribs
Abdomen
Respirations _____
Spine
Front Legs
Hind Legs
Paws (Pads, toes, claws)
Pulse _____
Tail _____

CAT'S NAME: _____

Date updated: _____

	At Rest	At Play
Pulse	_____	_____
Respiration	_____	_____
Temperature	_____	_____
Capillary Refill Time	_____	_____
Weight	_____	_____

Temperature (Normal = 100.4° F – 102.5° F)

Capillary Refill Time (2 seconds or less)

Average Heart Rate for Dogs and Cats

Species	Average Heart Rate
Cats	160 – 200 beats per minute
Small dogs	90 – 160 beats per minute
Medium to Large dogs	65 – 90 beats per minute

Average Respiration Rate for Dogs and Cats

Species	Average Respiration Rate
Cats and small dogs	20 – 40 breaths per minute
Medium to large dogs	10 – 30 breaths per minute

Please note: Very large dogs and/or geriatric animals may have slower respirations. Rule of thumb is the bigger and the older the dog or cat, the slower his pulse and respiration. The smaller and younger the animal, the faster their breathing and pulse.

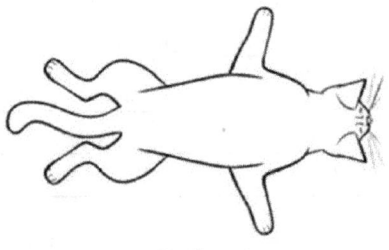

Sunny-dog Ink

Copyright 2015. Sunny-dog Ink.
www.SunnyDogInk.com

Healthy Cat Weight

Work with your veterinarian to make sure cat is a healthy weight. In general, you should be able to feel and/or see a cat's ribs through a thin layer of fat. An ideal weight is an important foundation for your cat's health and well-being.

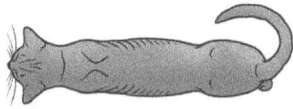

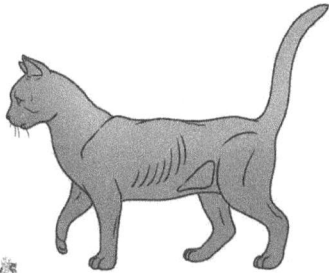

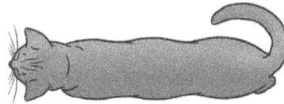

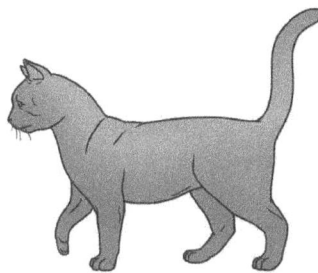

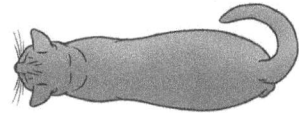

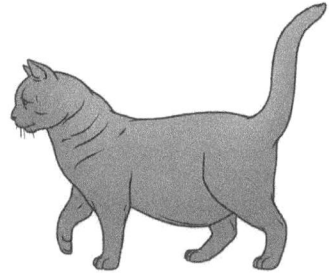

Thin to underweight, you will see or feel the ribs easily.

Ideal weight and a fit pet. Ribs can be felt, but not necessarily seen.

Ribs are not seen and can be difficult to feel.

Body Language Visual Chart

It's important to be able to understand your cat's body language.
Become familiar with their audible cues and visual clues.

Happy Cat

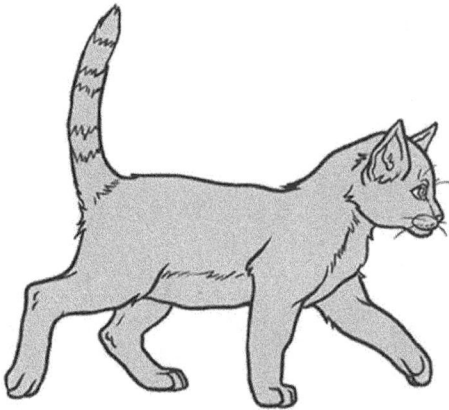

Sour Puss

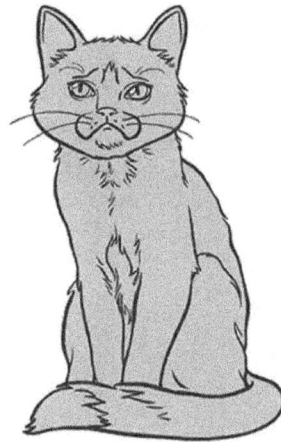

Scaredy Cat

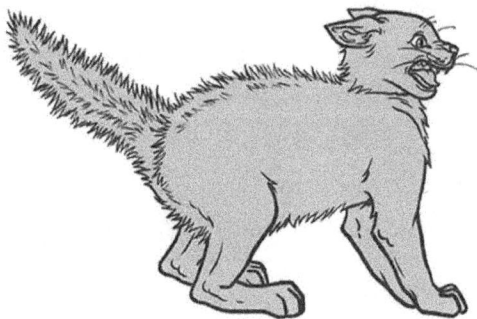

Sick Cat

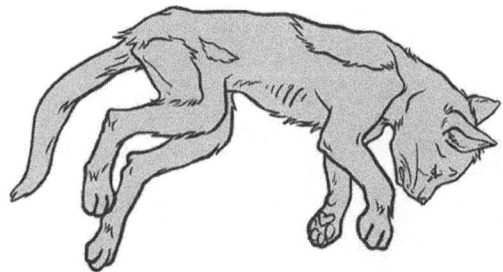

	Happy Cat	Sour Puss	Scaredy Cat	Sick Cat
Ears	Flat	Flat & Pressed Back Against Head	Pulled Back Against Head	To The Sides Or Any Abnormal Position
Eyes	Open & Bright	Pupils Narrow	Wide Open	Half Crossed
Hackles (Fur on the neck back)	Relaxed & Smooth Fur	Fluffed Up	Fluffed Up	Could Go Either Way
Tails	Relaxed or upright especially if the tip of the tail is curled can mean "howdy" from a cat . May lower front legs with butt in the air waggin tail with a "play bow".	Swishing with hair bristled or straight up like a bottle brush.	Tucked between legs or she'll bow with hair standing straight up.	Tucked Between Legs
Whiskers	Straight To The Side	Pulled Back Against Face	Forward Or Back	Pulled Forward Or Any Abnormal Position
Sounds	Gentle purring and meows from Cats.	Hissing or spitting, cats even chatter when frustrated.	Frightened cry to growing or hissing.	Cats may purr when comforted.
Rubbing Behavior	When cats rub against you or scratch objects they are leaving their scent saying you are their property; a sign of endearment			

Poisonous Plant List

Be diligent and always check to see if plants that your pets can interact with are safe. There are many plants that can be dangerous and have toxic effects on pets. This list is a starting point for pet parents and is not all-inclusive. This list includes some of the common plants and trees that can be poisonous or toxic to pets...

Aconite
African Evergreen
Alocasia
Amaryllis
American Holly
Angel's Trumpet
Anthurium
Apple Tree
Apricot Tree
Apple Leaf
Arrowgrass
Arrowhead vine
Asian Lily
Atropa Belladonna
Autmn Crocus
Azaleas
Baneberry
Beech Trees
Bird of Paradise
Bishop's Weed
Black Locust
BlueBonnet
Branching Ivy
Buckeye
Buttercup
Cardiac Glycosides

Castor Bean
Chinaberry Tree
Christmas Rose
Cowbane
Daffodils
Daphne
Day Lily
Dumbcane
Easter Lily
Elephant Ear
English Ivy
Fern Palm
Foxglove
Holly
Horse Chestnut
Hyacinth
Iris
Jerusalem Cherry
Jessamine
Jimson Weed
Lantana
Larkspur
Lily of the Valley
Lupine
Mayapple
Milkweed

Mistletoe
Monkshood
Morning Glory
Narcissus
Nightshade
Oleander
Oriental Lily
Periwinkle
Philodendron
Pokeweed
Poinsettia
Poison Hemlock
Rhododendron
Rhubard
Sago Palm
Shamrock
Skunk Cabbage
Star of Bethlehem
Sweet Pea
Tiger Lily
Tobacco
Water Hemlock
Wisteria
Yellow Oleander
Yew
Yucca

Common Poisons List

Be diligent and observe where and what your pets can interact with. There are many hazards and dangers that are constantly present in your pets lives. Preparation, awareness and avoidance are important for the safety of your pets. The following are some of the common poisons and hazards your pet may encounter:

Household Items:

Acetaminophen Products	Acids	Alkaline Products
Antibiotics	Antifreeze	Aromatherapy Oils
Aspirin	Batteries	Bleach
Carbon Monoxide	Cholecalciferol	Cigarettes
Cigars	Cleaners	Cocoa Mulch
Coins	De-icers	Deodorants
Deodorizers	Detergents	Dyes
E-Cigarettes	Fertilizers	Fireworks
Fuels	Fungicides	Herbacides
Gardening Products	Gardening Tools	Insecticides
Kerosene	Laxatives	Lead
Liquid Potpurri	Marijuana	Matches
Medications	Mothballs	Paintballs
Pesticides	Petroleum Products	Pine Oils
Plants	Prescription Medications	Rodenticides
Tobacco	Toys	Tools
Windshield Wiper Fluids	Zinc	

Foods & Consumables:

Alcohol	Bones	Bread Dough
Caffeine	Candy	Chocolate
Chicken Bones	Coffee	Fruit Pits & Seeds
Gum	Hops	Mushrooms
Onions	Rhubarb Leaves	Xylitol Products

There are many poisons and toxins that can impact your cat depending on their environment and access. Take a Cat's eye view of what is in the environment and take action to know what hazards exist and how you can reduce them.

MISSING PET

Missing Since: _____

Photo of Missing Pet Here	**Name:** _____
	Breed: _____
	Color: _____
	Distinguishing Features: _____
	_____
	_____
	Female / Male: _____
	Height / Length: _____
	Weight: _____
	Wearing ID: _____
	Wearing Collar: _____

If Seen/Found Please Contact: _____

_____

_____

Special Notes:

Your Cat's Vital Sign Record

Fill in these table so that you have a record of your cats' vital signs.
If you only have one cat, leave the lower record for later,
when your cat enters their senior years.

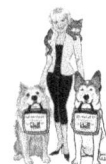

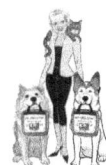

MY CAT'S VITALS

Pets Name			
	Normal	At Rest	After Play
Respiration	Cats: 20-40 inhalations per minute		
Pulse	Cats: 160 - 200 beats per minute		
Temperature	100.4° F - 102.5° F (38° C - 39.16° C)		
Weight			
Date			

Your Cat's Vital Sign Record

Fill in these table so that you have a record of your cats' vital signs.
If you only have one cat, leave the lower record for later,
when your cat enters their senior years.

MY CAT'S VITALS

Pets Name			
	Normal	At Rest	After Play
Respiration	Cats: 20-40 inhalations per minute		
Pulse	Cats: 160 - 200 beats per minute		
Temperature	100.4° F - 102.5° F (38° C - 39.16° C)		
Weight			
Date			

Pet Emergency Identification Card

In Case of emergency please make sure my pets are cared for.

Owner Name: _____   Phone: _____

Address: _____

Alternate Contact Info: _____

I have _____ pets at home.

Urgent Medical Concerns: _____

- -

Veterinarian: _____   Phone: _____

Pet #1: _____

Pet #2: _____

Pet #3: _____

Pet #4: _____

Pets At Home In Need:

Name: _____   Phone: _____

Name: _____   Phone: _____

Emergency Contact Information

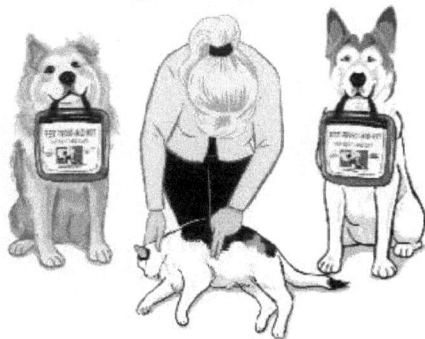

PET ALERT

Please Rescue our
Animal Family Members:

_____Dog(s)   _____Cat(s)   _____Bird(s)
_____Other (specify)_____

Emergency Contact: _____

_____

_____

_____

Thank you for caring!

Copyright ©2015. Sunny-dog Ink.
www.SunnyDogInk.com

Index

www.ingramcontent.com/pod-product-compliance
Lightning Source LLC
Chambersburg PA
CBHW081155020426
42333CB00020B/2513

9781949695106